Advanced nursing practice requires purposeful reasoning based on understanding theory as opposed to simply knowing about it. Understanding the intricate dance among quantitative and qualitative variables and their significance to the well-being of patients is dependent upon a constantly evolving theoretical base. As with most disciplines, nursing theory builds on a foundation of scientific evidence that provides the reliability and validity needed to provide safe care. However, human beings are more than science, and caring for them often necessitates we go where numbers cannot. Be it through logical adequacy or phenomenological exploration we build theory to guide our intercession with patients experiencing complex, often ethereal challenges. One such emerging theory is Dr. Maya Zumstein-Shaha's *The Omnipresence of Cancer*. In their forward-thinking text *A Theory of Cancer Care in Healthcare Settings*, Drs. Zumstein-Shaha and Cox demonstrate an understanding of the experience of cancer that is unparalleled. They deconstruct the experience concept by concept and reconstruct it into a whole that is greater than the sum of those parts – a blueprint that promises to guide the future of cancer care.

Professor Pamela Webber, *PhD, APRN, BC, FNP*
(Shenandoah University School of Health,
Winchester, Virginia, USA)

A Theory of Cancer Care in Healthcare Settings

This book provides healthcare professionals with a practice theory for the care and management of patients who have been diagnosed with cancer. It explores what patients experience and how healthcare professionals can assist them in dealing with their uncertainty and fear as well as planning for the future.

Unique to the book is its explication of the emerging theory, 'The Omnipresence of Cancer', which is set in the context of a discussion of earlier theories also concerned with cancer care. Chapters demonstrate how 'The Omnipresence of Cancer' has been developed, validated through research and being further tested in relation to cancer care. In particular, a chapter on philosophical reflections using theory to produce knowledge for practice is included. Each chapter provides essential background, a synthesis of the current state of knowledge, and practice examples associated with cancer care. The combination of theoretical reflection and practice examples is designed to promote comprehension and guidance on implementation of the theory, as well as recommendations for practice.

This book will be of significant interest to healthcare students and professionals working in the field of cancer care and oncology, particularly healthcare professionals working in advanced practice roles and nurse educators. It is also anticipated that professionals working in pastoral care, occupational therapy, social work, and radiography will be interested in this book.

Carol L. Cox is a Professor Emeritus at City University, London. She has been involved in teaching and research at various universities in the United Kingdom, Norway and the United States of America since 1987. Dr Cox practices as a nurse and instructs students and recent graduates (nursing, medicine, pharmaceutical and physiotherapy) at the Health and Hope Clinic in Pensacola, Florida, USA.

Maya Zumstein-Shaha has been a Professor at the University of Applied Sciences Health in Berne since October 1, 2017. She has been a senior lecturer at the University of Lausanne, Switzerland. Prof Zumstein-Shaha teaches nursing theory and also supervises students studying at the masters and doctoral levels. Prof Zumstein-Shaha also serves as member on the National Advisory Commission on Biomedical Ethics CNE.

Routledge Research in Nursing

Pragmatic Children's Nursing
A theory for children and their childhoods
Duncan C. Randall

Forthcoming titles:

A Theory of Cancer Care in Healthcare Settings
Edited by Carol L. Cox and Maya Zumstein-Shaha

A Theory of Cancer Care in Healthcare Settings

Edited by Carol L. Cox and
Maya Zumstein-Shaha

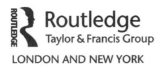

Routledge
Taylor & Francis Group

LONDON AND NEW YORK

First published 2018
by Routledge
2 Park Square, Milton Park, Abingdon, Oxon OX14 4RN

and by Routledge
605 Third Avenue, New York, NY 10017

First issued in paperback 2021

Routledge is an imprint of the Taylor & Francis Group, an informa business

British Library Cataloguing-in-Publication Data
A catalogue record for this book is available from the British Library

Library of Congress Cataloging-in-Publication Data
A catalog record for this book has been requested

ISBN 13: 978-0-367-34151-0 (pbk)
ISBN 13: 978-1-138-64376-5 (hbk)

Typeset in Times New Roman
by Apex CoVantage, LLC

Contents

Preface

This monograph addressing Cancer Care in an Emerging Theory for Health Care Professionals was initiated at the request of patients and families affected by colorectal cancer. The chapters presented in this book have been constructed from research conducted over the past ten years. Most of the research undertaken has been within the domain of nursing; however, within the past few years, the research has extended to embrace allied health professionals' work. Subsequently, this book encompasses perspectives and strategies for caring for cancer patients underpinned by the theory *The Omnipresence of Cancer*, which is an original theory discovered by Maya Shaha as part of her doctoral research. The chapters present case examples to assist the health care professional discern contextual approaches for the provision of cancer care.

Chapter 1 presents an introduction to theory, theory formation for practice and the essence of the underlying theory that substantiates the necessity for the chapters that follow. This chapter familiarizes the reader with the understanding that theory, be it generated through deduction, induction or construction is subject to hypothesis formation and testing. Original sources have been referenced to highlight the complex history of nursing knowledge associated with nursing theory. Perspectives drawn from eminent authors writing over the past 40 years inform the reader regarding the historical nature of theory in practice. Once this background has been provided, a distinction is made between the context of discovery and the context of justification which relates to the relevance of constructing the theory of *The Omnipresence of Cancer* (Shaha and Cox, 2003).

Chapter 2 presents phenomenology and theory formation, with reference to health care. Phenomenology and theory as usually understood are discussed, and phenomenology as a body of *descriptive* knowledge is presented. The phenomenological method, which inevitably involves *epoché*, a suspension of certain kinds of judgment on certain kinds of things adds a dimension for the foundation of phenomenological investigations. A parallel is drawn which lays the foundation for understanding the processes involved in the development of the theory *The Omnipresence of Cancer* and its implications in health care.

Chapter 3 presents a systematic review of existing theories in cancer care. While grand theories are referenced in theoretical frameworks applied to cancer, including their influence on middle-range theories developed for cancer, specific application of theory to cancer has proliferated in the last decade through the emergence of more middle-range theories to guide research, practice, and education. Areas of theoretical focus are discussed. In the past, the largest population of interest involved the patient. However, increasing focus on palliative care has expanded the population of interest to include family and non-family caregivers. Relationship issues specifically related to cancer treatment, illness trajectories, and survivorship as well as end-of-life management have also become more important lately. Emerging conceptual models related to cancer care are examined. The systematic review of existing theories highlights the need for further study of the cancer illness trajectory, with focus on social, psychological and spiritual care.

Chapter 4 presents a full explication of the theory of *The Omnipresence of Cancer*. It addresses two concepts, *Transitoriness* and *Uncertainty*, and how these affect cancer care from the perspective of the patient, family and health care professional. The theory *The Omnipresence of Cancer* is described. Background knowledge associated with cancer is addressed. Patients' reactions to a diagnosis of cancer and the necessity for developing theory is presented. A case example that presents the theory, *The Omnipresence of Cancer*, which was derived from research conducted amongst patients with a diagnosis of colorectal cancer is presented to promote a more comprehensive understanding of the theory and its constructs. *The Omnipresence of Cancer*, as a theory, is to facilitate an understanding of having been diagnosed with cancer and its effect on the ontology[1] of human existence multi-dimensionally.

Chapter 5 presents ethical dimensions associated with caring for cancer patients and their families within the constructs of the theory: *The Omnipresence of Cancer*. The chapter indicates that selecting a theory for practice is influenced by the selectors' values, beliefs and attitudes. It is therefore necessary to identify these elements in a theory. Based on these findings, the theory's acceptability by the health professionals and the clinical practice where it is supposed to be used, can be determined. Uncovering the basic values and beliefs of a theory are shown to help to identify mechanisms for essentially creating an ethically sensitive practice and provision of such care to patients and their families. Once this is established, caring can then be negotiated in the clinical area and relevant and adequate interventions can be identified, developed and implemented in the respective clinical practice.

Chapter 6 presents the first sub-construct of the theory *The Omnipresence of Cancer*, which is Transitoriness. Instrument development for the purpose of conducting research is discussed with reference as to how the health care professional can use the instrument in practice to inform patient and family care. It is shown that the development of the instrument meets the current expectations of support for the psychosocial needs of patients diagnosed with cancer. The instrument offers to health professionals a working tool as much as theoretical support. It helps in the understanding of cancer patients' experiences as well as an evaluation of the finitude of life. The construct of Transitoriness highlights the need to educate health professionals about the finitude of life and its related experience.

Chapter 7 presents coping strategies that may be employed with cancer patients and their families. The theory *The Omnipresence of Cancer* offers a solid frame of reference for the studies presented in this monograph, thereby documenting the processes and mechanisms that favor the integration of cancer's omnipresence into the life of persons concerned. A vignette of a clinical situation demonstrates the relevance of this theory for use in clinical practice in oncology. It is shown that with implementation of this theory, health professionals are guided to better understand the cancer patients' experience. Subsequently, tailored interventions can be developed and implemented, which allow patients to develop and use appropriate and unique coping strategies.

Chapter 8 presents the second sub-construct, Uncertainty, experienced amongst cancer patients and their families. It demonstrates that Uncertainty constitutes an important aspect of a patient's cancer trajectory. The chapter recommends the integration of regular and systematic assessments from the moment of the diagnosis onward. Uncertainty as an experience is present in almost all types of cancer, independent of gender, age and level of education. Health care providers are presently described as not possessing sufficient information on the experience of Uncertainty to provide effective and supportive care to patients with a cancer diagnosis. The theory *The Omnipresence of Cancer* can assist practitioners in identifying the importance of Uncertainty within the cancer trajectory and support the development of adequate interventions for patients and their families as well as other health care professionals.

Chapter 9 presents spirituality in health care provision. This chapter postulates that nursing and, in general, health care as practice disciplines has yet to find their way in relation to discerning an evidence base for the provision of spiritual care. It has been shown that although nursing is credited with initially having nurtured the interest in spirituality and its implications for spiritual care, there is profound criticism of its poorly constructed scholarship including conceptual confusion and lack of evidence to substantiate its practice recommendations and claims associated with spiritual care. It is evident that nurses and health care professionals, in general, are unable to substantiate their practice base in regard to spirituality and do not have a definitive evidence base for the practice of spiritual care, particularly within the context of end of life care. *The Omnipresence of Cancer*, as a theory, is shown to be for nurses and health care professionals, in general, the beginning of an evidence base for the delivery of spiritual care.

Chapter 10 presents the epilogue of the monograph, which summarizes the key components for caring for a patient and family experiencing the ravages of cancer. It delineates the key associations of Chapters 1 through 9 and reinforces the need for implementation of the theory *The Omnipresence of Cancer.*

Note

1 Ontology means specification of a conceptualization.

Contributors

Anne E. Belcher, PhD, RN, ANEF, FAAN

Associate Professor (Retired) Johns Hopkins School of Nursing, Baltimore, Maryland; Associate Professor, Sidney Kimmel Comprehensive Cancer Centre, Baltimore, Maryland; Associate Professor (Clinical), Johns Hopkins University School of Education, Baltimore, Maryland.

Chapter 3. Existing theories in cancer care

Carol L. Cox, PhD, MA, MA, MSc, PG Dip, PGC, BSc (Hons), FD, RN, FHEA

Professor Emeritus City University London; Clinic Manager, Health and Hope Clinics, Pensacola, Florida.

Chapter 1. An introduction to theory: theory formation for practice (featuring *The Omnipresence of Cancer*)

Chapter 4. Theory of *The Omnipresence of Cancer*, including two concepts: uncertainty and transitoriness

Chapter 8. Uncertainty in cancer patients

Chapter 9. Spirituality in healthcare provision

Chapter 10. Epilogue

Maria-Goretti Da Rocha Rodrigues, RN, MScN, PhD (c)

Lecturer, University of Applied Sciences and Arts, Western Switzerland, School of Nursing, Geneva, Switzerland.

Chapter 7. Coping strategies in cancer patients

Sandra Gaillard Desmedt, RN, MScN

Vice-Dean post graduate education, University of Applied Sciences and Arts, Western Switzerland, School of Nursing, La Source, Lausanne, Switzerland.

Chapter 7. Coping strategies in cancer patients

Alfonse Grieder, PhD, BA (Hons)

Professor Emeritus, City University London.

Chapter 2. Phenomenology and theory formation, with reference to health care

Daniel Kelly, PhD, MSc, PGCE, BSc, RN, FRCN, FRSA

Professor, School of Healthcare Sciences, Cardiff University, Eastgate House, Cardiff, Wales; Royal College of Nursing Chair of Nursing Research & Director of Research and Innovation, Royal College of Nursing, London, England.

Chapter 8. Uncertainty in cancer patients

Maya Zumstein-Shaha, PhD, MSc, BSc (Hons), RN

Professor, Senior Lecturer, University Institute of Higher Education and Research in Healthcare, Faculty of Biology and Medicine, University of Lausanne, Switzerland.

Chapter 3. Existing theories in cancer care

Chapter 4. Theory of *The Omnipresence of Cancer*, including two concepts: uncertainty and transitoriness

Chapter 5. Ethical dimensions of the theory: *The Omnipresence of Cancer*

Chapter 6. Transitoriness: instrument development

Chapter 8. Uncertainty in cancer patients

Chapter 10. Epilogue

Kirsi Talman, PhD, MSc, PGCE, RN

Senior Lecturer, Clinical Nursing and Emergency Care, Metropolia University of Applied Sciences, Metropolia, Finland.

Chapter 8. Uncertainty in cancer patients

Gina Tavares Sobral, RN, MScN, CNS

Centre for hereditary haematologic diseases, University Medical Centre Lausanne, Switzerland.

Chapter 6. Transitoriness: instrument development

Verena Tschudin, PhD, MA, BSc (Hons), RN

Visiting Senior Fellow, University of Surrey, Surrey, England.

Chapter 5. Ethical dimensions of the theory: *The Omnipresence of Cancer*

Jennifer Wenzel Song, PhD, RN, CCM, FAAN

Associate Professor, Johns Hopkins School of Nursing, Baltimore, Maryland; Associate Professor, Johns Hopkins School of Medicine, Baltimore, Maryland; Associate Professor, Sidney Kimmel Comprehensive Cancer Center, Baltimore, Maryland.

Chapter 3. Existing theories in cancer care

1 An introduction to theory

Theory formation for practice

C. Cox

Introduction

Theory, be it generated through deduction, induction or construction, is subject to hypothesis formation and testing. Martha Rogers (1970) indicated in her publication *An Introduction to the Theoretical Basis of Nursing* that theory describes, explains and predicts. Some years later, Walker and Avant (1988) indicated theory also controls practice. Further on in nursing's evolution, Johnson and Webber (2001) indicated that theory moves from prediction to influencing practice and therefore controls practice. Throughout the history of nursing, theories have informed the practice of nursing science through rigorous research. The purpose of this chapter is to explicate theory formation for practice. Wherever possible, original sources will be referenced to highlight the complex history of nursing knowledge associated with nursing theory. Perspectives drawn from eminent authors writing over the past 40 years will inform the reader regarding the historical nature of theory in practice. Once this background has been provided, a distinction will be made between the context of discovery and the context of justification which relates to the relevance of constructing the theory of *The Omnipresence of Cancer* (Shaha and Cox, 2003), which is relevant in the practice of cancer nursing.

Background

Theory formation for practice

It was postulated by Chinn and Jacobs (now Kramer) that "[t]he development of theory is the most crucial task facing nursing today" (1978: 1). It is postulated that this perspective holds true as practice evolves in the 21st century. Certainly, within the realm of informing practice, before theory can be developed, a sound understanding of the levels of theory and its concepts/constructs is required (Johnson and Webber, 2001). Practice is based on knowledge that has a sound scientific basis. The development and testing of theories trough research provides the scientific knowledge required for practice (Johnson and Webber, 2001). During the 20th and 21st centuries, the foundations of theory development have been discerned. These begin with levels of theory development.

Literature has explicated four levels of theory development. The first level is meta-theory, which has its focus on philosophical and methodological questions (Refer to Chapter 2 for an in-depth discussion of philosophical perspectives and phenomenology.). For example, *The Omnipresence of Cancer* (Shaha and Cox, 2003) as a theory for cancer nursing practice is based on the philosophical phenomenological perspective of Martin Heidegger's (1962) *Being and Time*.

The second level is grand theory, which consists of broad perspectives which form a model or framework for the construction of the third level which is middle-range theory and subsequently the fourth level, which is practice or situation-specific theory. Middle-range theory is less abstract than grand theory and fills the gap between grand theory and practice or situation-specific theory. Practice or situation-specific theory, as it may be termed, provides prescriptions for practice. For example, Martha Rogers's theory, *Nursing, A Science of Unitary Man (The Science of Unitary Human Beings)* (Rogers, 1980) inspired the development of Margaret Newman's theory on *Health As Expanding Consciousness* (Newman, 1986) and Rosemary Parse's *Man, Living Health: A Theory of Nursing* (Parse, 1981). Newman's theory and Parse's theory began as middle-range theories which have subsequently evolved into grand theories. Each of their theories, in turn, has inspired considerable research which has spawned other middle-range theories that inform perspectives in practice. Table 1.1 provides the levels of theory relevant to nursing.

Walker and Avant (1988) indicated meta-theory focuses on broad issues related to theory in nursing and in the main does not produce any grand, middle-range or practice theories. The issues considered at the level of meta-theory include, and in many circumstances, are not limited to, "(1) analyzing the purpose and kind of theory needed in nursing, (2) proposing and critiquing sources and methods of theory development in nursing, and (3) proposing the criteria most suited for evaluating theory in nursing" (Walker and Avant, 1988: 5). It is evident from Walker's and Avant's (1988, 2011) viewpoint that at the meta-theoretical level, debate is extant within the domain of philosophy. Literature articulating perspectives on

Table 1.1 Levels of theory

Meta Theory
Grand Theory (Conceptual Models/Frameworks)
Middle Range Theory
Practice Theory – Situation-Specific Theory

Legend: Table adapted from Fawcett, J. and Walker, L. and Avant, K. (Fawcett, 1995; Walker and Avant, 1988)

meta-theory focuses on examinations of the meaning of nursing as a practice discipline and the identification of nursing as a science and profession.

Grand theories are broad, abstract narratives that present perspectives on goals to be achieved and the structure of nursing practice (Chinn and Jacobs, 1978; Chinn and Kramer, 1999, 2008, 2015; Fawcett, 1995, 2000; Walker and Avant, 1988, 2011). These broad and abstract theories provide global perspectives for practice, education and research. Walker and Avant indicated in 1988 that grand theories are limited as they presently exist and, because of their generality and abstractness, are untestable. This perspective is valid today.

The process of theorizing involves the construction of concepts and statements. Concepts and statements are derived from analysis, synthesis and derivation. The process of analysis and construction of concepts and statements must be relatively concrete in order to engage in theory testing. Construct construction is derived, in the main, through research. To engage in theory testing at the grand theory level means that the narrative within grand theories would need to be concrete rather than vague and the interrelationships between concepts would have to be delineated with sufficient precision so that predications (associated with practice) could be undertaken (Walker and Avant, 2011). Theoretical testing, therefore, must begin at the middle-range theory level wherein constructs and statements are concrete enough to be tested (Jacox, 1974). Some examples of grand theories are shown in Table 1.2.

Table 1.2 Examples of grand theories

Date of publication	Grand theory	Author
1952	Interpersonal Relations in Nursing	Peplau
1961	The Dynamic Nurse-Patient Relationship	Orlando
1964	Clinical Nursing: A Helping Art	Wiedenbach
1966	The Nature of Nursing	Henderson
1967	The Four Conservation Principles of Nursing	Levine
1968	Determinants of the Nurse-Patient Relationship	Ujhley
1970	An Introduction to the Theoretical Basis of Nursing	Rogers
1971	Toward a Theory of Nursing	King
1971	Nursing: Concepts of Practice	Orem
1971	Interpersonal Aspects of Nursing	Travelbee
1974	The Betty Neuman Health-Care Systems Model	Neuman
1976	Introduction to Nursing: An Adaptation Model	Roy
1979	Toward a Theory of Health	Newman
1980	The Behavioral System Model for Nursing	Johnson
1981	Man-Living-Health	Parse
1981	A Theory for Nursing: Systems, Concepts, Process	King
1985	Nursing: Human Science and Human Caring	Watson
1986	Health as Expanding Consciousness	Newman
1992	The Human Becoming Theory	Parse

Legend: Adapted from Fawcett, J. (Fawcett, 1995)

Middle-range theory is a workable level of theory (Jacox, 1974). At middle-range theory level, variables inherent in the theory are limited, as well as the theory's abstract nature (scope). Middle-range theory is generalizable enough to apply to a variety of nursing practices/settings but concrete enough to be tested within a variety of nursing practices/settings. For example, in the middle-range theory *The Omnipresence of Cancer*, the construct of *Uncertainty* can apply to a variety of nursing practices. Uncertainty emerges whenever a patient must undergo a new procedure such as the initiation of chemotherapy (*Will this cure my cancer?*) or a surgical procedure (*Will I be able to walk again after this surgery?*) or during a mental health consultation (*If I talk to this nurse and tell her about my problems, will I feel better?*). These are merely a few examples of nursing practice areas in which *Uncertainty* must be addressed by the nurse. In relation to research and practice, middle-range theories contain some of the conceptual perspectives of grand theories but provide concrete propositions which can be tested.

Practice theory, or situation-specific theory, emerges from middle-range theory. Jacox (1974) indicated that practice theory has a goal and prescriptions for action that will achieve the goal. Table 1.3 demonstrates the progression of theory through research. At the practice theory level, for example, controls are situated in policies, procedures, guidelines and protocols. Practice theory is "theory that says given this nursing goal (producing some desired change or effect in the patient's condition), these are the actions the nurse must take to meet the goal (produce the change). For example, a nursing goal may be to prevent a postoperative patient form becoming hyponatremic. Nursing practice theory states that, to prevent hyponatremia, a particular set of actions must be taken" (Jacox, 1974: 10).

Distinction between the context of discovery and justification

It may be argued that the distinction between the context of discovery and justification is one of substance. Discovery often involves reflection on a philosophical perspective, which then becomes integrated, forming the foundation of a grand

Table 1.3 The progression of theory through research

Theory:	*Describes*	*Explains*	*Predicts*	*Controls*
Research:	Qualitative Descriptive Quantitative Descriptive	Qualitative Explanatory Quantitative Correlational	Quantitative: Experimental	Policies Procedures Guidelines/Protocols

Legend: Adapted from Fawcett, J. and Downs, F. and Walker, L and Avant, K. (Fawcett, and Downs, 1992; Walker and Avant, 1988)

theory. This process in and of itself is one of creativity. Fawcett (1995) indicated in her publication on conceptual models that the focus and content of a conceptual model reflects its philosophical claims. This then also becomes apparent in its emergent middle-range theory, which subsequently informs practice theory. It is also extant in the development of middle-range theory which has not yet evolved into grand theory or has any goal to evolve into grand theory. Justification, on the other hand, presents the reasonable grounds for a particular philosophical perspective. It provides an argument that substantiates formulation of the theory in accordance with a philosophical perspective.

Concepts inherent in theory may be discovered through induction or deduction. Observations may be made either in the process of or in practice or through reflection on a philosophical perspective, such as Martin Heidegger's (1962) *Being and Time* that forms the philosophical foundation of the middle-range theory *The Omnipresence of Cancer*. Construction of theory is distinct from its evaluation. In the generation of a theory, it is constructed through discovery and then evaluated to discern the theory's strengths and weaknesses. The process of evaluation involves research: testing the theory's propositions within the context of practice. It is also evaluated by comparing the theory with criteria such as explication of the theory's origins, comprehensiveness of content and logical consistency. "Prematurely imposing the standards and methods used in theory evaluation upon theory generation can lead to rejection of a promising theory and stifling the creative process" (Walker and Avant, 1988: 14). For more information on the processes involved in the evaluation of theory refer to Fawcett's (1995) publication on the *Analysis and Evaluation of Conceptual Models in Nursing*. The aforementioned have relevance in relation to the theory of *The Omnipresence of Cancer* (Shaha and Cox, 2003). The *Omnipresence of Cancer* was discovered in the process of studying Martin Heidegger's (1962) *Being and Time* and discovering how its premises could inform nursing practice within the context of cancer nursing.

Discussion

The Omnipresence of Cancer: constructed through research

The Omnipresence of Cancer, as a middle-range theory, began as a doctoral research project. The project addressed the phenomena of living with a diagnosis of colorectal cancer. Rationale for undertaking the research was because a need had been identified in practice to describe the experience of living with a diagnosis of colorectal cancer and what this means to an individual and its relevance for informing and controlling nursing practice. In order to discern the theory, a phenomenological study was undertaken based on Heidegger's (1962) philosophy as presented in his seminal work *Being and Time*. The project involved exploratory qualitative descriptive first level research. To explore the lived experience

of colorectal cancer, seven patients diagnosed with colorectal cancer were inter-
viewed over a time span of 13 months. This provided an opportunity to discover
the lived experience of the patients being diagnosed and undergoing treatment
for their disease. Patients participating in the study were recruited from three
Swiss hospitals. Data were analyzed by following Colaizzi's eight-step process
as cited in Haase (1987: 66–67). Analysis identified one main category: 'The
Omnipresence of Cancer' and two sub-categories: 'Towards Authentic Dasein'
(Towards Authentic Being) and 'Mapping out the Future'. The research demonstrated that having received a diagnosis of cancer means an individual is faced
with the potential of lifelong illness and death. The research further found that
individuals experiencing this disease feel stigmatized by the diagnosis and are
classified as belonging to an illness group. Furthermore, the research determined
that individuals who have been diagnosed with colorectal cancer need to talk with
health care professionals about their experiences and concerns. It is important that
in-depth discussions occur between patients and health care professionals so that
the patient's questions and uncertainties may be addressed. Within the confines of
the theory, it is apparent that health care professionals must become educated and
have a sound understanding of mechanisms that can facilitate the development of
coping strategies which patients and their families can employ.

Conclusion

In this chapter, elements of theory generation were presented. The chapter explicated theory formation for practice. Wherever possible, original sources were referenced to highlight the complex history of nursing knowledge associated with
nursing theory. Perspectives drawn from eminent authors writing over the past
40 years informed the reader regarding the historical nature of theory in practice,
levels of theory and the progression of theory through research. A distinction was
made between the context of discovery and the context of justification which
relates to the construction of the theory *The Omnipresence of Cancer* (Shaha and
Cox, 2003). *The Omnipresence of Cancer*, as a theory, is evolving. It is presently
undergoing quantitative testing to further discern mechanisms that will control
nursing practice and subsequently facilitate the improvement of the patient experience when undergoing diagnosis and treatment of cancer.

References

Chinn, P. L. and Jacobs, M. K. 1978. A model for theory development in nursing. *Advances
    in Nursing Science*, 1(1), 1–11.
Chinn, P. L. and Kramer, M. K. 1999. *Theory Construction in Nursing Theory and Nursing
    Integrated Knowledge Development*, fifth edition. St. Louis: Mosby.

Chinn, P. L. and Kramer, M. K. 2008. *Theory and Nursing Integrated Knowledge Development*, eighth edition. St. Louis: Mosby.

Chinn, P. L. and Kramer, M. K. 2015. *Knowledge Development in Nursing, Theory and Process*, ninth edition. St. Louis: Mosby.

Fawcett, J. 1995. *Analysis and Evaluation of Conceptual Models of Nursing*, third edition, Philadelphia: F. A. Davis Company.

Fawcett, J. 2000. *Analysis and Evaluation of Contemporary Nursing Knowledge: Nursing Models and Theories*. Philadelphia: F. A. Davis Company.

Fawcett, J. and Downs, F. S. 1992. *The Relationship of Theory and Research*, second edition. Philadelphia: F. A. Davis Company.

Haase, J. E. 1987. Components of courage in chronically ill adolescents: a phenomenological study. *Advances in Nursing Science*, 9(1), 64–80.

Heidegger, M. 1962. *Being and Time*. Oxford: Basil Blackwell Ltd.

Jacox, A. K. 1974. Theory construction in nursing: an overview. *Nursing Research*, 23(1), 4–13.

Johnson, B. and Webber, P. 2001. *An Introduction to Theory and Reasoning in Nursing*. Philadelphia: Lippincott.

Newman, M. A. 1986. *Health as Expanding Consciousness*. St. Louis: C. V. Mosby Company.

Parse, R. R. 1981. *Man, Living Health: A Theory of Nursing*. New York: John Wiley.

Rogers, M. E. 1970. *An Introduction to the Theoretical Basis of Nursing*. Philadelphia: F. W. Davis Company.

Rogers, M. E. 1980. Nursing: a science of unitary man. In J. P. Reihl and C. Roy (eds.), *Conceptual Models for Nursing Practice*, second edition. New York: Appleton-Century-Crofts, pp. 329–37.

Shaha, M. and Cox, C. L. 2003. The omnipresence of cancer. *European Journal of Oncology*, 7(3), 191–6.

Walker, L. O. and Avant, K. C. 1988. *Strategies for Theory Construction in Nursing*, second edition. Connecticut: Appleton and Lange.

Walker, L. O. and Avant, K. C. 2011. *Strategies for Theory Construction in Nursing*, fifth edition. New York: Pearson.

2 Phenomenology and theory formation, with reference to health care

A. Grieder

Introduction

Phenomenology and theory, as usually understood, seem methodologically opposed to one another. A phenomenology is a body of *descriptive* knowledge. It is the result of applying a method whose aim is to describe what or how things are, describe them without recourse to theorising and in a manner that is as unprejudiced as possible. Usually, the problematic condition is added that what is described has to be *directly given*. But what is directly given, i.e., given as itself and without any mediation whatever? However, one cannot simply disregard this condition. What is described should at least be experienced as directly as possible, e.g., without relying on hearsay, experimentation (unless it is simple and transparent), theoretical assumptions, or causal analysis. Hence, a phenomenological method inevitably involves an *epoché*, a suspension of certain kinds of judgement on certain kinds of things. Admittedly, most of our sciences would be considerably impoverished if they were reduced to phenomenologies. On the other hand, phenomenological investigations are called for when and where speculation gets out of hand and theories lose their contact with concrete experience, and also where new fields of experience and research have to be opened up. In this chapter, phenomenology and theory formation with reference to health care will be presented. A parallel with be drawn which lays the foundation for understanding the processes involved in the development of the theory *The Omnipresence of Cancer* and its implications in health care.

Background

Types of phenomenology

There are various types of phenomenology, scientific and non-scientific, philosophical and non-philosophical, empirical and non-empirical. Some are concerned with natural, some with mental or social phenomena, and some are so different from each another that one hesitates to bring them all under this one heading 'phenomenology'. A phenomenology worthy of its name will of course amount to more than a jumble of descriptions and will systematically explore a range of phenomena. The phenomenological approach was already practiced in Greek antiquity, surprisingly perhaps, in view of their flair for bold ideas and speculative thought. The Hippocratic Writings (dating mostly from the 5th or 4th centuries BC) include medical case studies and reports such as the following: "A woman of the household of Pantimides took a fever the first day after a miscarriage. Tongue was parched: thirst, nausea and insomnia, bowels disordered, the stools being thin, copious and raw. – Second day: rigors, high fever, much purgation; did not sleep. – Third day: pains more intense. – Fourth day: became delirious. Seventh day: died. – The bowels were relaxed throughout; the stools being watery, thin, raw and voluminous; urine little and thin" (Lloyd, 1978: 119). Here we have an empirical and truly phenomenological account, based upon direct observation not too different from everyday observation, just more refined, more focused and supported by some expertise in these matters, an account free of speculation, theorising and causal explanation. An epoché is clearly in place.

By contrast, to theorise is to think up principles and more or less abstract ideas, establish logical relations between them and use them to link up, explain or predict things. A theory, then, is a body of general and coherent knowledge claims that is related to certain particulars, in such a manner that the theoretical assertions can be confirmed or disconfirmed by statements about some of these particulars. In a sense, of course, every phenomenology is concerned with the general, for to describe something is to apply *general terms* to it, to describe it as being of such and such a kind. Thus, while the above Hippocratic account concerns a particular person and her illness, it has to make use of terms such as 'miscarriage', 'fever', 'nausea', 'bowels', each of which could also be applied to other particulars in other situations. The decisive point is that a theory has to do more than bringing particulars under general concepts: it must enable one to explain or at least systematically correlate them. A complication arises, however. Assume the Greek author of the above report used such descriptions to establish a typology of common diseases. He might then, having observed the initial phases of a person's illness, use his observations to predict the likely course and type of the disease. His phenomenology could then claim to be a low-level theory. The borderline between theoretical and descriptive investigations is not as clear-cut as might be assumed, a difficulty we shall return to.

Phenomenology according to Husserl, Jaspers and Heidegger

Phenomenology did not start with Husserl, but with Husserl and the Phenomenological Movement he initiated. It took a new turn (or rather several new turns) and had in due course a considerable impact not only on philosophy but also on the human studies generally. H. Spiegelberg (1978), *The Phenomenological Movement* in two volumes, is still the best available account of this Movement; see esp. the sections on Husserl and Heidegger in Volume 1. Also recommendable is R.C. Solomon (1972), *From Rationalism to Existentialism. The Existentialists and their 19th Century Background*, Chapters 5 and 6. Husserl's aim was a philosophical phenomenology culminating in a transcendental phenomenology. However, with it was associated a phenomenological psychology, which can serve as a kind of prolegomenon to it. In the following, I shall be concentrating on this phenomenological psychology, as it is more easily accessible than transcendental phenomenology and more directly related to the issues of health care. Note that readers looking for Husserlian introductory texts may find the following helpful: E. Husserl (1950), *The Idea of Phenomenology*; *Phenomenology*, in Husserl's (1971) *Encyclopedia Britannica* article (1927), *Husserl, Shorter Works* (McCormick and Elliston, 1981) and *Author's Preface* in *E. Husserl (1962) Ideas. General Introduction to Pure Phenomenology* (Boyce Gibson, 1962).

Psychology as commonly practised concerns itself with the psychical (perception, memory, emotions etc.) as bound up with the human body and its biological conditions. Relying on external observation and experiment it attempts to gain knowledge of our mental life. According to Husserl, this psychology is grounded in our natural attitude, hence primarily concerned with outwardly accessible facts and unable to come to terms with what should be its proper subject matter: the psychical itself. He writes: "The ubiquitous fundamental trait of this psychology is to set aside any direct and pure analysis of consciousness [. . .] in favour of indirect fixations of all psychological or psychologically relevant facts, having a sense that is at least superficially understandable without such an analysis of consciousness, at best an outwardly understandable sense" (Husserl, 1965: 92). It operates with crude class concepts of perception, imagination, recognition, expectation, forgetting etc., but in Husserl's view, its very methodology prevents it from clarifying these concepts.

In order to remedy this defect, Husserl proposes a *pure, eidetic psychology* (PEP, for short), which is meant to serve as a basis for empirical psychology. As a pure psychology, it abstracts from all physical or biological facts and features; as an eidetic psychology, it concerns itself with the descriptions of essential structures of consciousness. Thus, to realise PEP a twofold epoché, a suspension of the natural attitude is required. The psychical as we commonly take it has to be reduced, stripped of its factual, natural-objectivistic sense. Husserl did not reject (as is sometimes falsely claimed) empirical and experimental psychology; rather, his objective was to provide it with a proper basis, so that what is commonly obscured and marginalised, namely the essence of the purely psychical, can be brought to light.

The basic character of consciousness is its directedness, i.e., that it is consciousness-of . . . that the experiences ('Erlebnisse') constituting it are experiences of something. This fundamental feature Husserl calls *intentionality.* Any item of consciousness has its intentional object, which is the object *as given in that consciousness*, the intended object. Phenomenological description is concerned with both, the essential structure of the experienced (the noema) as well as that of the correlated experiencing (noesis) in which the intended object is given. It describes the various essential forms of this noetic-noematic correlation, e.g., in perceptual consciousness, memory, imagination. Husserl writes: "All that bears the title 'consciousness-of' and that 'has' a 'meaning', 'intends' something 'objective', which latter [. . .] permits being described as something 'immanently objective', 'intended as such' and intended in one or another mode of intending. That one can here investigate and make statements, and do so on the basis of evidence, adapting oneself to the sense of this sphere of 'experience', is absolutely evident" (Husserl, 1952: 109); (the quotation marks around some of the terms indicate that these must be understood with the epoché in mind.) According to Husserl, the essential structures of consciousness can be directly given in a kind of intuition or ideation ('Wesensschau'). There is some doubt, however, about what precisely this intuition of essences amounts to and to what extent structures of consciousness can be clearly and distinctly revealed in this manner.[1] As the essential structures, PEP is supposed to reveal are general structures of all consciousness and can be exemplified in actual individual experiences, PEP could, with some justification, be called a low-level theory.[2]

PEP did not make the impact on modern psychology Husserl had hoped for. However, at least his insistence that there is more to psychology than observing and theorising about outwardly manifest behaviour soon found an echo in Jaspers's pyscho-pathological phenomenology. He too saw himself confronted with a one-sided scientific practice, a psychiatry for which all mental illnesses were defects of the brain and nervous system. He writes: "My own investigations as well as my reflections about what was being said and done in psychiatry had led me on tracks which were new at that time. Philosophers gave me the impetus for two essential steps. As method, I adopted Husserl's phenomenology which, in its beginnings, he called descriptive psychology; I retained it although I rejected its further development to insight into essences ('Wesensschau'). It proved to be possible and fruitful to describe the inner experiences of patients as phenomena of consciousness. Not only hallucinations, but also delusions, modes of ego-consciousness, and emotions could, on the basis of the patients' own descriptions, be described so clearly that they became recognizable with certainty in other cases. Phenomenology became a method for research" (Jaspers, 1981: 18). The first thing, then, was to understand what the patient's experiences are, then describe and delimit them, compare and order them according to their affinities, and provide a suitable terminology for them. What had to be described, i.e., patients' actual concrete experiences, is not given in some direct 'Wesensschau' but has to be established by *emphatic understanding*, assisted by various indirect means (e.g., observation of patients' behaviour, use of their self-descriptions etc.) (Jaspers, 1963, 1968). An epoché is obviously applied (although Jaspers does not seem to use the term): all genetic and causal considerations, all theorising, any inclusion of factors that are not 'in the subjects' consciousness' have to be excluded. Jaspers had no intention of adopting the whole of Husserl's phenomenology. It is a single idea in it that spurred him on: the idea of a purely descriptive approach to consciousness.

Heidegger was the most influential and outstanding among Husserl's followers. His main work *Being and Time* (Heidegger, 1962) is an ontological inquiry, an inquiry into being or the sense of being. To answer this question Heidegger thought it necessary to probe, first of all, into the being of 'Dasein', i.e., the human being. This preliminary inquiry, called fundamental ontology, is the only published part of the project whose main question, the 'question of being', is only partly answered. The phenomena Heidegger focused upon are of an ontological character, but he also referred to ontic phenomena, and sometimes it is not entirely clear whether what is commented on is of an ontological or of an ontic nature. (This important distinction between the ontic and the ontological we shall shortly return to.) While Husserl was mainly concerned with the essential structures of consciousness, above all its intentionality, Heidegger's phenomenology is an interpretation of Dasein's being and meant to reveal the ontological structure of human existence and being-in-the world. In this sense, at least it is an *existential phenomenology*. The following – inevitably sketchy – comments are based on *Being and Time* (Heidegger's later philosophy cannot be considered here). The abbreviation BT refers to this work, and SZ to the 8th ed. of M. Heidegger, *Sein und Zeit* (originally published in 1927). Roughly speaking, his inquiry proceeds in three stages. First, Dasein's basic ontological condition of *being-in-the world* is dealt with as well as a number of Dasein's ontological traits, the so-called *existentialia* (to be distinguished from the categories, i.e., the ontological determinations of entities not of the kind of Dasein). These are then shown to be founded in the embracing structure of *Care*. In a third step, Dasein's being is interpreted with regard to its *temporality*.

In its everyday world, Dasein encounters other entities, other Dasein, but also the ready-to-hands (utensils, equipment such as hammers, tables etc.) and what is present-at-hand (entities – e.g., scientific objects – encountered in a manner detached from the immediate everyday concerns). Readiness-to-hand and presence-at-hand are two modes of being of entities that are not of the kind of Dasein. Utensils are linked up in a network of significance and in-order-to connections (e.g., hammers in order to hit nails, nails to fix boards, boards to make tables, and so on) relating back to Dasein. Other Dasein is encountered primarily in one's work-world and along with the equipment used: "they [i.e., others] are encountered as what they are; they *are* what they do" (Heidegger, 1962: BT 153, 163; Heidegger, 1927: SZ 117, 126). In this way, Dasein comes under the sway of the others: "The Self of everyday Dasein is the *they-self*", an inauthentic and average self that tends to fall in line with the others and the way things are publicly interpreted and done, a self 'levelled down', while being preoccupied with maintaining spurious differences between itself and the others. *Fallenness* is what characterises this everyday existence (Heidegger, 1962: BT 166–7, 220–1; Heidegger, 1927: SZ 128–9, 175–6).

Its own being is *disclosed* to Dasein, and so is worldly being. Such disclosure need not be full disclosure and tends to go together with partial concealment. Heidegger (1962) distinguishes three basic modes of disclosure: *attunement* (also called *state-of-mind*), *understanding* and *discourse*. Attunement, ontically apparent as moods, unveils to Dasein, prior to all cognition, that it is and has to shoulder its burdensome existence; it also enables Dasein to direct itself towards anything at all and to discern what 'matters' to it in the world (Heidegger, 1962: BT 174–6; Heidegger, 1927: SZ 153–7). Fear and dread (Angst) are modes of attunement, but while fear is fear of something within the world, dread concerns Dasein's being-in-the-world as such; fallenness is rooted in dread (Heidegger, 1962: BT 179, 230–1, 233; Heidegger, 1927: SZ 140, 186, 188). Understanding discloses to Dasein its potentiality for being, i.e., what it is capable of, and thus opens up leeways for being in the world (Heidegger, 1962: BT 184–5; Heidegger, 1927: SZ 144–5). Projecting itself forward in this manner, Dasein is said to be 'ahead of itself'. Sight, circumspection, knowing, interpreting are all grounded in understanding (Heidegger, 1962: BT 186–7; Heidegger, 1927: SZ 146–7). The rich section devoted to *discourse* goes far beyond the usual philosophy of language. Discourse is an articulation of one's being-in-the-world; being-with-others is discursive, being silent an essential possibility of discourse and listening a way of opening up to other Dasein (Heidegger, 1962: BT 204, 206–8; Heidegger, 1927: SZ 161, 163–4). To the extent that the *they-self* dominates Dasein's being, the three main modes of disclosure degenerate into curiosity, ambiguity and chatter, which characterise *fallenness* and *inauthenticity*. Finally, all these existentialia are brought together in the embracing structure of *Care:* Dasein's being ahead-of itself-already-in (the world)-as-being-alongside (entities encountered in the world) (Heidegger, 1962: BT 237; Heidegger, 1927: SZ 192). Care is then interpreted in terms of Dasein's temporality and *finitude* ('being towards death'), and existential temporality (as distinct from clock time and the series of 'nows' – called 'vulgar time') described as a threefold movement, with the future as the guiding mode. (Heidegger, 1962: BT; Heidegger, 1927: SZ sections 65 and 66) – Heidegger's approach takes us beyond Husserl's phenomenology of consciousness and beyond the traditional idea of the 'animal rationale', let alone the various theological, metaphysical and behaviouristic conceptions of 'man' put forward in western philosophy. These perspectives are relevant to understanding the theory *The Omnipresence of Cancer.*

Discussion

On the use of phenomenology in theory formation

A full and adequate analysis of this topic could fill many pages. I shall have to restrict myself to some aspects of it. To begin with, what is a theory? There are different kinds of theories, some empirical, some non-empirical (e.g., mathematical, metaphysical, normative). Scientific empirical theories are such that they can be intersubjectively confirmed or disconfirmed by observation or experiment. Some theories are quantitative-nomological (i.e., contain general laws of the type which we find, e.g., in the physical sciences), while others, especially in the social and human studies, where such laws are difficult to come by, are not. There appears to be agreement that theories should at least be consistent, involve some general claims about a range of particulars and be of use to link these up, coordinate and explain them.

The processes of theory formation are so varied that all that can be done here is to draw attention to a few, often recurring, types. The widely held, view that theories are arrived at through an extensive inductive process, i.e., starting with the exploration of a wide range of particulars and then moving on to the generalisation of the results, is in need of qualification. Obviously, some knowledge of the particulars is needed in order to establish a theory about them. However, the history of the sciences provides many examples where theories are arrived at not by first establishing large collections of facts, but by accounting for (explaining, linking up) a relatively small number of them that are considered particularly relevant. There may be subject areas, however, where a thorough phenomenology of the range of particulars is called for before promising theoretical proposals can be made. Often, theories are developed by modifying or merging already existing theories. Theories in adjacent fields may provide models to follow. Sometimes, work in quite different fields may suggest fruitful ideas or novel perspectives for one's own research.

Of special interest, in this context, is the role played by philosophical ideas in theory formation. It is well known that, e.g., Pythagorean and Platonic ideas, ancient atomism, the Cartesian ontology and Francis Bacon's (1902) *Novum Organum* influenced the course of the physical sciences. But how can a philosophy be of use to an empirical science? The knowledge claims of an empirical science must be intersubjectively testable, confirmed and hitherto unrefuted. Philosophies can hardly be expected to satisfy this requirement. Furthermore, they seem at least as fallible as scientific knowledge, and it is therefore a dubious enterprise to search for some unshakable philosophical foundation to underpin scientific claims. An empirical science has to stand up to empirical tests; in this sense, it has to 'stand on its own feet'. However, this does not rule out the possibility that scientific work may be guided by philosophical ideas. After all, a science is also an activity; there is more to it than the body of its knowledge claims.

Before a scientific theory can be established or radically changed, the range and nature of the things to be accounted for has to be roughly circumscribed, the field of research articulated in a preliminary manner. In both these respects philosophical ideas can play a fruitful role. Heidegger has seen this clearly: "Basic concepts determine the way in which we get an understanding beforehand of the area of subject-matter underlying all the objects a science takes as its theme, and all the positive investigation is guided by this understanding" (Heidegger, 1962: BT 30; Heidegger, 1927: SZ 10). Further: "And although research may always lean towards this positive approach, its real progress comes not so much from collecting results and storing them away in 'manuals' as from inquiring into the ways in which each particular area is basically constituted [. . .] The real 'movement' of the sciences takes place when their basic concepts undergo a more or less radical revision which is transparent to itself" (Heidegger, 1962: BT 29; Heidegger, 1927: SZ 9). While it has to be admitted that the sciences are partly determined by factors that are not strictly scientific ('positive'), and that these may include philosophical orientations, one can hardly share Heidegger's confidence that philosophy is able to provide them with some definite ontological foundation.

An empirical phenomenology such as the Hippocratic one mentioned previously in this chapter, may provide useful knowledge of particulars from which one may inductively ascend to tentative generalisations or by means of which generalisations may be tested. However, Husserl's and Heidegger's phenomenologies are not of that type. The former is concerned with essences rather than particulars; the latter with ontological rather than ontical matters. Husserl clearly distinguished between empirical and eidetic inquiries and pointed out that the eidos must not be identified with some empirical generality as the latter depends on a finite sample of cases from which it is extracted, while the eidos refers to an ideal infinity of cases. Heidegger makes a similar point regarding the ontical and ontological: "As compared with this ontical interpretation, the existential-ontological Interpretation is not, let us say, merely an ontical generalisation which is theoretical in character. [. . .] The generalisation is rather one that is *ontological and a priori.* What it has in view is not a set of ontical properties which constantly keep emerging, but a state of Being which is already underlying in every case [. . .]" (Heidegger, 1962: BT 243–4; Heidegger, 1927: SZ 199). An empirical study is neither eidetic nor ontological. A thorough analysis of its relationship to eidetic phenomenology and ontology cannot be provided here. In short, if the eidetic assertions of PEP and Heidegger's ontological claims are of any use in empirical inquiries, they must at least be approximately exemplifiable in the empirical or ontical domain. They may do more than that and open up new domains and perspectives of empirical research by drawing attention to phenomena not seen or not sufficiently appreciated before.

The legacy of the Phenomenological Movement is twofold. It was inspired by the Husserlian call 'Back to the things themselves!', away from speculative thought, system-building and discursive procedures, in order to attend to what is properly within our grasp, given in such a manner that it can be described in some detail. This approach was then applied to bring to light structures of consciousness and everyday human existence which had hitherto attracted little attention and should be of much interest to the social and human studies. Thus, Husserl's idea of a descriptive psychology focusing on consciousness itself enabled Jaspers to break away from a psychopathology that was almost exclusively based on the outwardly observable and on theories based on the natural sciences. In psychology and in the social and human studies a similar situation had arisen. Positivistically inclined methodologies derived from the natural sciences exerted their influence. They tended to marginalise the 'subjective' dimension of human life, yet were presented as the only scientific way forward. To correct this one-sidedness, directives are needed for both observation and theory that bring the neglected 'subjective' phenomena to the fore. This does not mean that those objectivistic approaches should be entirely dismissed; it simply means that there is much more to humans, their experience and comportment than what can be observed and theoretically dealt with in the manner of the natural sciences. The Phenomenological Movement offered a variety of perspectives that enable researchers to come to terms with this other, 'subjective' reality. – Medical care is a case in point. It clearly has to use methods of the natural sciences or akin to those of the natural sciences. Yet it has to take note of two basic facts: (i) that good care has to approach patients as human beings – not just bodies, and (ii) that it depends to some extent on how carers and patients collaborate and communicate, and on their attitudes towards each other. So the 'subjective' dimension has to be probed into. But here intersubjective testability is more problematic, the scope of quantification and measurement much more restricted and the measurable often not what is most relevant. Hence the temptation to marginalise this dimension of medical care.

Towards a Heideggerian perspective in theory formation and caring

It is not difficult to see why the Heideggerian ontological phenomenology of Dasein has its attractions for many who try to come to terms with the nature and practice of health care. He put forward what is welcomed as an *original holistic* conception of human beings which – contrary to the traditionally recommended 'objectivistic approach', puts the emphasis on *how humans experience themselves and their world* and face up to what an Italian author aptly called *'il mestiere di vivere'*. Some qualifications are needed, however, and we shall see that there is also a crucial, perhaps surprising omission in his fundamental ontology. I can only make a few tentative suggestions as to how Heideggerian existential phenomenology may be of use for theory formation in this field.

Regarding the 'holistic' character, *Being and Time* (Heidegger, 1962) does certainly do justice to several basic features of being human: e.g., being in and inseparable from the world, emotionally tuning in with it, having a practical understanding of it and an awareness of possibilities towards which one may project oneself, being with others and mostly falling in line with them. These and other ontological traits are then brought together and linked up in the embracing structure of Care. Occasionally, at philosophy conferences, persons working in the social services or medical institutions told me that Heidegger's philosophy was of interest to them 'because it addresses the problem of care'. In a sense, it does, but 'Care' is, of course, an ontological term, whereas what they referred to was care as we usually understand it and which is, from the Heideggerian point of view, some ontical correlate of the existentiale *solicitude*. The psychiatrist Binswanger (1942) thought he had to draw attention to the phenomenon of love in order to compensate for a certain one-sidedness in the account of Care in *Being and Time*. He too seems to have misunderstood what Heidegger meant, namely that Care is an ontological condition that determines our being whether we comport ourselves lovingly or unlovingly, whether we care or don't care (Binswanger, 1942).[3]

There is one condition of being human that is of major importance in health care and which Heidegger hardly goes into: embodiment. To be sure, he presupposes it. For how could there be readiness-to-hand without hands, being-towards-death without embodiment? Yet a phenomenology of how we live our bodies is missing in *Being and Time*. Had it been Heidegger's intention to give us a philosophical anthropology, one may rightly expect such a phenomenology. He had no such intention, however; rather, his objective was to elaborate an ontology of Dasein to the extent that it is required in order to answer the question of being. By contrast, a theory of medical care has to come to terms with a double perspective: with the body as experienced by the patient himself/herself, and with the body as the object of medical knowledge and medical treatment. Carers have to take account of both these perspectives. Connected with that omission is another feature of Heidegger's approach: it focuses on average Dasein. It is left to the reader to puzzle out whether or to what extent his existential phenomenology is relevant to our understanding of early childhood, of the lives of the severely mentally handicapped, or of those who have to cope with prolonged extreme suffering. Finally, health care needs norms – norms of good care, an issue that falls outside the scope of Heidegger's project. It should be clear, therefore, that *Being and Time*, whatever useful suggestions it may provide for a theory of medical health care, cannot provide a *sufficient* philosophical basis for it.

Let us briefly consider some of Heidegger's existentialia that may be of particular interest in this context. To determine their ontical manifestations and significance requires in most cases an interpretation which goes beyond the scope of *Being and Time*, although Heidegger does sometimes comment on them. It is up to those engaged in health care to attempt such interpretations such as in the process which has been done in developing the theory, *The Omnipresence of Cancer*. Here are a few hints in this direction. "What we indicate *ontologically* by the term 'state of mind' is *ontically* the most familiar and everyday sort of thing; our mood, our Being-attuned" (Heidegger, 1962: BT 172; Heidegger, 1927: SZ 134). Moods are not just fleeting and more or less accidental emotional states. Having primordial disclosure function, they co-determine an individual's situation in a very basic manner. With regard to health care this would suggest that patients are not only thinking and perceiving beings but through their moods disclosed to themselves and in touch with the world around them; that moods set the tone for all the interactions between carers and those they care for; and that depending on their moods patients will react differently to the carers and the care received, face up differently to their illnesses and chances of recovery. In short, health care has to take care of patients' moods. *Understanding* discloses one's potentiality-for-being, possibilities towards which one may project oneself. Humans are essentially self-projecting, and understanding is therefore closely connected with the future and temporality (Heidegger, 1962: BT 182–4, 385–9; Heidegger, 1927: SZ142–4, 336–339). This existentiale should draw our attention to the ontical fact that one's awareness of what one is able to do or not able to do plays a decisive role in one's life (Refer to the theory, *The Omnipresence of Cancer* for clarification as to how this has been addressed within the theory as an example.). Thus, a patient may have to be made aware that certain possibilities are within his/her reach or, alternatively, that possibilities he/she wants to hang on to have become unrealisable and that life has to be reorientated. A patient's response to medical care may be crucially determined by how he/she 'sees' the future. The *finitude* of Dasein figures as a central issue in *Being and Time*; "death is a possibility-of-Being", Heidegger says, and it is one's *ownmost* possibility (Heidegger, 1962: BT 294; Heidegger, 1927: SZ 250). Words that should make medical personnel reflect on, indeed question the view that problems regarding the treatment of the terminally ill have to be decided mainly or even exclusively on 'objective medical grounds'. *Solicitude* is an existentiale founded in Care and Being-with-others and structurally related to state-of-mind, understanding and discourse. Nursing of sick bodies is mentioned as one ontical manifestation of solicitude. As all Dasein is characterised by fallenness, deficient modes of solicitude (such as passing one another or taking others as if they were present-at-hands) prevail in average everyday being-with (Heidegger, 1962: BT 153–63, 158; Heidegger, 1927: SZ 117–25, 121). Solicitude can take two extreme forms. Somebody may leap in for somebody else: "This kind of solicitude takes over for the Other that with which he is to concern himself. The Other is thus thrown out of his own position; he steps back so that afterwards, when the matter has been attended to, he can take it over as something finished and at his disposal or disburden himself of it completely. In such solicitude the Other can become one who is dominated and dependent, even if this domination is a tacit one and remains hidden from him" (Heidegger, 1962: BT 158; Heidegger, 1927: SZ 122). With this form, Heidegger contrasts another one: solicitude as leaping ahead of the other "not in order to take away his 'care' but rather to give it back to him authentically [. . .] it helps the Other to become transparent to himself *in* his care and to become *free for* it" (Heidegger, 1962: BT 158–9; Heidegger, 1927: SZ 122). Such help clearly presupposes an understanding of the other, of *his* moods, *his* awareness of what he is able to be and do. While some philosophers (e.g., Wilhelm Dilthey, 1833–1911) stressed the importance of empathic understanding, empathy is in Heidegger's view a derivative phenomenon, grounded in Dasein's primordial understanding of others, but helpful in order to counter the prevailing deficient forms of solicitude.

Conclusion

It is an outstanding feature of the Husserlian, Heideggerian and other phenomenologies that they probe into the 'subjective' dimension of being human and describe various structures underlying the ways we experience ourselves and the world. The human 'subject' is seen as essentially open to the world, and in some manner or other most of those structures concern this openness. Some (like Husserl) focus on consciousness and its intentionality, others (like Heidegger) on being-in-the-world. Heidegger's (1962) existential phenomenology as elaborated in *Being and Time* is of course not concerned with health care as such; it is an ontological treatise. His term 'Care' refers to a basic ontological condition of Dasein and means something quite different from what we normally call 'care'. Theories in or of health care are at least partly of empirical character (but may involve normative elements as well). Operating on the empirical or (as Heidegger would say) ontical level they have to comply with the requirement of intersubjective testability. The ontological structures Heidegger describes may indeed help to elucidate the practice of health care and suggest guidelines for theory formation in this field. But they can only provide suggestions, i.e., suggest empirical generalisations as correlates of Heideggerian existentialia. In the end, such generalisations have to stand up to observational tests, and it would be naïve to think that an ontology could provide unshakable foundations for them.

Notes

1 Note that some of Husserl's descriptions of internal time-consciousness and of picture-consciousness go beyond what my intuition is able to ascertain clearly and distinctly; to me, they seem to involve hypothetical elements, possibly suggested by some intuitive hunches – their intersubjective testability and hence their scientific status – which Husserl was keen to underline appears to some extent doubtful.
2 Husserl does occasionally use the term 'theory' for his phenomenological descriptions, e.g., in I*deen III* (1952: 140).
3 See L. Binswanger, *Grundformen und Erkenntnis menschlichen Daseins*, Zurich, 1942, and Binswanger's comments on his 'misinterpretation' in the preface to the 3rd and 4th editions, as well as part 1, chapter 1, section A, IV d. – Compare M. Heidegger, *Zollikoner Seminare. Protokolle, Gespräche, Briefe* (ed. M. Boss), Frankfurt, 1987. English

version: M. Heidegger, *Zollikon Seminars: Protocols, Conversations, Letters* (ed. M. Boss) (trs. R. Askay and F. Mayr), Evanston, IL, 2001; in particular pp. 150–2, 157, 236–8, 253. See also M. Heidegger, 'On Adequate Understanding of Daseinsanalysis', *Humanistic Psychologist*, 16 (1988); contains on pp. 75–98 several relevant excerpts from the Seminars (trs. M. Eldred)).

References

Bacon, Sir Francis. 1902. *Novum Organum*, ed. by M. A. Joseph Devey. New York: P.F. Collier. Available at: http://oll.libertyfund.org/titles/1432 Originally published in 1620 [Accessed February 28, 2017].

Binswanger, L. 1936/1942. *Grundformen und Erkenntnis menschlichen Daseins*. Zurich: Freuds Auffassung.

Heidegger, M. 1927. *Sein und Zeit*. Frankfurt AM Main: Vittorio Klostermann.

Heidegger, M. 1927/1996. *Sein und Zeit* (Martin Heidegger's magnum opus *Being and Time* originally published in 1927). New York: State University Press.

Heidegger, M. 1962. *Being and Time*, trans. by J. Macquarrie and E. Robinson. Oxford: Basil Blackwell Ltd, reprint of the first edition of 1962.

Heidegger, M. 1987. *Zollikoner Seminare. Protokolle, Gespräche, Briefe*, ed. by M. Boss. Frankfurt am Main: Vittorio Klostermann.

Heidegger, M. 1987/2001. *Zollikon Seminars: Protocols, Conversations, Letters*, ed. by M. Boss, English Version, trans. by R. Askay and F. Mayr. Evanston, IL: Springer, pp. 150–2, 157, 236–8, 253.

Heidegger, M. 1988. On adequate understanding of daseinsanalysis. *Humanistic Psychologist*, 16(1), 75–98 (Translation M. Eldred).

Husserl, E. 1927. Phenomenology, Encyclopedia Britannica. *The Journal of the British Society for Phenomenology*, 2 (1971).

Husserl, E. 1950. *The Idea of Phenomenology*, trans. by W. P. Alstonand and G. Nakhnikian. The Hague, Netherlands: Springer Publishers.

Husserl, E. 1952. *Ideen III*, 'Nachwort'. The Hague, Netherlands: Martinus Nijhoff, pp. 109–40.

Husserl, E. 1962. Author's preface. In E. Husserl (ed.), *Ideas: General Introduction to Pure Phenomenology*, trans. by W. R. Boyce Gibson. New York: Routledge.

Husserl, E. 1965. *Phenomenology and the Crisis of Philosophy*, ed. by Q. Lauer. New York: Harper, p. 92.

Husserl, E. 1981. *Husserl: Shorter Works*, eds. by P. McCormick and F. A. Elliston. Notre Dame: University of Notre Dame Press.

Jaspers, K. 1913/1963. *General Psychopathology*, trans. by J. Hoenig and M. W. Hamilton. Manchester: Manchester University Press, Part 1, Chapter 1.

Jaspers, K. 1968. The phenomenological approach in psychopathology. *British Journal for Psychiatry*, 114, 1313–23.

Jaspers, K. 1981. Philosophical autobiography. In P. A. Schilpp (ed.), *The Philosophy of Karl Jaspers*. La Salle, IL: Springer, p. 18.

Lloyd, G. E. R., ed. 1978. *Hippocratic Writings*. Hamondsworth, Middlesex: Peguin Books, p. 119.

Solomon, R. C. 1972. *From Rationalism to Existentialism. The Existentialists and their 19th Century Background*. London: Humanities/Harvester Press.

Spiegelberg, H. 1978. *The Phenomenological Movement*, 2 Volumes. The Hague: Martinus Nijhoff Publishers.

Bibliography

Binswanger, L. 1942. *Grundformen und Erkenntnis menschlichen Daseins.* Zurich: Max Niehans Verlag.

Heidegger, M. 1927. *Sein und Zeit.* Frankfurt am Main: Vittorio Klostermann

Heidegger, M. 1988. On adequate understanding of daseinsanalysis. *The Humanistic Psychologist,* 16, 75–98.

Heidegger, M. and Boss, M. 1987. *Zollikoner Seminare: Protokolle, Gespräche, Briefe.* Frankfurt am Main: Vittorio Klostermann

Heidegger, M. and Boss, M. 2001. *Zollikon Seminars: Protocols, Conversations, Letters.* Evanston, IL: Northwestern University Press.

Heidegger, M., MacQuarrie, J. P. U. T. S. N. Y. and Robinson, E. S. 1962. *Being and Time,* trans. by John Macquarrie and Edward Robinson, First English edition. London: SCM Press.

Hippocrates, Lloyd, G. E. R., Chadwick, J. and Mann, W. N. 1978. *Hippocratic Writings.* Harmondsworth: Penguin.

Husserl, E. 1930. Nachwort zu meinen "Ideen zu einer reinen Phänomenologie und phänomenologischen Philosophie". *Jahrbuch für Philosophie Und Phänomenologische Forschung,* 11, 1–22.

Husserl, E. 1971. "Phenomenology" Edmund Husserl's article for the Encyclopaedia Britannica (1927): New complete translation by Richard E. Palmer. *Journal of the British Society for Phenomenology,* 2, 77–90.

Husserl, E., Alston, W. P. and Nakhnikian, G. 1950. *The Idea of Phenomenology,* trans. by William P. Alston and George Nakhnikian. Introduction by G. Nakhnikian. The Hague: Martinus Nijhoff.

Husserl, E., Elliston, F. A. and McCormick, P. 1981. *Husserl: Shorter Works.* Notre Dame, IN: University of Notre Dame Press; Brighton: Harvester Press.

Husserl, E. and Gibson, W. R. B. 1962. *Ideas: General Introduction to Pure Phenomenology,* [S.l.]: Collier-MacMillan, 1962 (1972).

Husserl, E. and Lauer, J. Q. 1965. *Phenomenology and the Crisis of Philosophy: Philosophy as Rigorous Science and Philosophy and the Crisis of European Man,* trans. with Notes and an Introduction by Quentin Lauer. New York: Harper & Row.

Jaspers, K. 1968. The phenomenological approach in psychopathology. *British Journal for Psychiatry,* 114, 1313–1323.

Jaspers, K., Hamilton, M. W. and Hoenig, J. 1963. *General Psychopathology,* trans. by J. Hoenig and Marian W. Hamilton. Manchester: Manchester University Press.

Schilpp, P. A. and Jaspers, K. 1981. *The Philosophy of Karl Jaspers.* La Salle, IL: Open Court; London: Distributed by Eurospan.

Solomon, R. C. 1992. *From Rationalism to Existentialism: The Existentialists and their Nineteenth-Century Backgrounds.* Lanham, MD: Littlefield Adams Quality Paperbacks.

Spiegelberg, H. 1978. *The Phenomenological Movement a Historical Introduction,* Volumes 1 and 2. The Hague: Martinus Nijoff.

3 Existing theories in cancer care

*A. E. Belcher, J. Wenzel Song and
M. Zumstein-Shaha*

Introduction

Scientific disciplines aim at systematically producing and collecting knowledge about a specific area of inquiry. The knowledge produced in such a way is considered reliable and specific to the respective discipline (Rodgers, 2005; Meleis, 2012). These tenets apply to nursing as well as other scientific disciplines such as palliative care. For nursing, it is essential the knowledge that is produced scientifically also includes application to the clinical domain.

Nursing's body of knowledge is organized into various units, which are called "conceptual models", "theories" or "concepts". The encompassing element in nursing that demarcates the discipline is called metaparadigm and consists of four concepts, which are person, environment, health and nursing (Fawcett and Desanto-Madeya, 2013; Smith and Liehr, 2014). These four metaparadigm concepts are represented in the different units of organized knowledge, i.e., conceptual models, theories or concepts.

The development of "conceptual models" in nursing started in the 1940s. This type of organized knowledge is considered to be more abstract than "theories" or "concepts" (Fawcett and Desanto-Madeya, 2013). Often, personal experiences of the theorists, in combination with research findings and in-depth reflective processes, have contributed to the development of conceptual models. Drawing on conceptual models, the development of knowledge in a given discipline is guided as well as education.

Theories constitute the next level of abstraction in nursing. This term also denotes a specific type of knowledge that is again divided into three levels of abstraction. In nursing, there are grand theories, middle-range theories and micro or situation-specific theories. Each one of these terms relates to the level of abstraction of a theory and indicates the potential of translating it into practice (Smith and Liehr, 2014; Fawcett and Desanto-Madeya, 2013; McEwen and Wills, 2007). Grand theories often have a similar way of being developed as conceptual models. Research findings are paired with personal experiences of the theorist and in-depth reflective thought processes eventually lead to the construction of a grand theory. This type of knowledge is also used as a guide to the discipline, to knowledge development and education. For the development of middle-range theories, about five different ways have been identified. These include the development of theories by drawing on existing nursing and non-nursing theories or by drawing on problems that have arisen in practice, which are subsequently studied in more detail (Smith and Liehr, 2014; Shaha, 2016). (Note that within the context of this monograph, *The Omnipresence of Cancer* as a middle-range theory was drawn from the problem of supporting cancer patients in practice.)

Middle-range theories are considered less abstract than conceptual models or grand theories. Their implementation in nursing practice is considered straighter forward, thereby providing much-needed innovation and promoting nursing practice (Smith and Liehr, 2014; Peterson and Bredow, 2009; Roy and Roy Adaptation Association, 2014). It is therefore important for nursing science to develop nursing theories with a medium scope, also to move practice forward. Theories with a micro range and specific to situations often have a close tie to clinical practice and emerge from quantitative or qualitative studies (Meleis, 2012; Im, 2011). Although they are even more concrete than middle-range theories, their specific scope limits the applicability in practice. However, middle-range and situation-specific theories are considered important stepping stones in the development of prescriptive practice theories as suggested by (Dickoff and James, 1968b; Dickoff and James, 1968a).

Conceptual models and grand theories direct the discipline from which they have emerged in the selection of pertinent phenomena that need to be studied, in guiding research and education and in providing information for management. Nursing's conceptual models and grand theories constitute the first theory-building elements and have been essential in bringing the discipline forward (Alligood, 2013; Fawcett and Desanto-Madeya, 2013).

Both conceptual models and theories are constituted of concepts, assumptions and propositions. Generally, conceptual models and grand theories include more than two concepts. These concepts at least have a label and in some cases there

Table 3.1 Overview of the ways of developing middle-range theories

Way of development	Example
Inductively by drawing on research	*The Omnipresence of Cancer* by Shaha
Deductively from research and practice implementation of grand theories or conceptual models	Theory of Adaptation to Chronic Pain by Dunn based on Roy's Adaptation Model
Combining existing nursing and non-nursing theories	Pain: a balance between analgesia and side-effects by Good
Deriving from theories from other disciplines	Theory of self-efficacy by Resnick based on social cognitive theory by Bandura
Deriving from practice guidelines and standards that are based on research	Theory of the Peaceful End of Life by Ruland and Moore

Legend: Table adapted from Liehr and Smith (1999).

exist theoretical or even operational definitions. Middle-range and situation-specific theories are expected to include at least one to two concepts. In contrast to more abstract theories, the concepts of middle-range and situation-specific theories are labeled and possess theoretical and operational definitions. It is also probable that their characteristics are identified. However, no specific number of concepts is indicated that are needed to form a theory.

Concepts are considered abstractions of real-life phenomena that consist of a given label, characteristics or attributes and defined outcomes (Morse et al., 1996; Cutcliffe and McKenna, 2005). Such constructions can remain on their own or put in conjunction with each other through assumptions and propositions. Assumptions propose the underlying philosophical influence. Propositions provide linkages between the concepts. These linkages are either derived from the underlying assumptions or from research. Concepts can be considered on their own. When linked together, concepts are the building blocks of theories. The assumptions provide, in these cases, essential information on the prerequisites of the theory, and propositions disclose potential areas of inquiry related to the theory or hypotheses for testing (McEwen and Wills, 2007).

The proposed knowledge classification is used in nursing and may not be shared by other scientific disciplines. However, this classification can be used to identify the level of knowledge abstraction, thereby identifying gaps in the literature. In addition, the metaparadigm concepts of person, environment, health and nursing are also specific to nursing. Exploring the presence of these metaparadigm concepts in the respective theories can help in identifying their importance for the nursing discipline and practice.

For the purpose of this chapter, the classification including conceptual models, theories – i.e., grand, middle and situation-specific – concepts and empirical indicators will be used to identify the level of abstraction of subsequently presented theories. In addition, the major concepts of any theory presented below will be briefly introduced, and it will be identified whether the presented theory addresses issues of finitude of life. By providing these aspects of the subsequently introduced theories, it will be possible to provide an overview of existing theories of palliative care that also addresses issues of finitude of life.

Background

In this chapter, existing theories in cancer and palliative care will be described and reviewed. To date, a number of theories are being used in various healthcare settings, notably also in cancer and palliative care. However, the contribution of these theories to cancer and palliative care, in particular, has yet to be determined. When theories are being used in these contexts, the application is rarely systematic or is not based on an informed decision making process.

A systematic review of existing theories in cancer and palliative care will provide an overview as well as indicate basic aspects that will help oncology practitioners, educators and other actors in healthcare to choose the most suitable theory.

An overview of theories addressing palliative care issues has rarely been provided in the literature. Only Dobrina et al. (2014) have conducted a systematic review and have proposed three theories, namely a theory by Desbiens et al. (2012), a theory on the unitary caring by Reed (2010), and a theory of transitions into palliative care by Murray (2007). In nursing, the well-known theories such as published by Alligood (2013), Fawcett and Desanto-Madeya (2013), Meleis (2012), Smith and Liehr (2014) or others, specific theories addressing palliative care are not identified. In addition, the palliative care domain is interdisciplinary and theories may need to take the variable perspective into account. Hence, it seems pertinent to review the current literature again in order to identify more recent additions to this field. Therefore, a systematic literature review was conducted in Pubmed/Medline and CINAHL between 1994 and 2016. The table found in the Appendix to this chapter provides an overview of the MesH-terms used, the relevant publications as well as the theories identified.

Discussion

A total of two conceptual models, six grand theories, five middle-range theories, one situation-specific theory and two concepts were identified in this search. Among the two conceptual models, hope, from the discipline of psychology, is presented. We provide a model of relevant middle-range theories and fuller descriptions of identified theories with direct relevance to cancer care which we believe will be pertinent to readers.

Grand theories of relevance to cancer care

Dorothea Orem's self-care theory

Orem referred to her conceptual model as the Self-Care Deficit Theory (Fawcett and Desanto-Madeya, 2013; Orem et al., 2003; Orem et al., 1995). Refer to Figure 3.1 in the Appendix in this chapter, which delineates Orem's theory. The core concept is entitled self-care, which corresponds with "health-related activities performed by individuals on their own behalf to maintain life, health and well-being" (Desbiens et al., 2012: 2115). Orem proposed a classification of nursing situations that comprise seven groups, with the final group being that of life-limiting illness; the focus is on quality of life that is seriously affected, until it reaches the point where life can no longer continue. The focus then shifts to maintaining the person's comfort at the end-of-life. Nursing is provided to patients

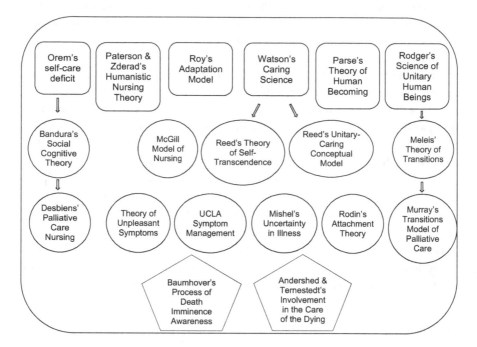

Figure 3.1 Overview of systematic review results

Legend: Chart visualizing the results of the systematic review of the nursing theories. The squares denote grand theories, the rounds relate to middle range theories, and pentagons refer to situation-specific theories. Arrows point to a general connection between the respective theories. The concepts (hope, liminality, mortality, palliative care, survivorship, and symptom management) have not been added to this figure.

with self-care deficits and to their families to help patients satisfy their self-care demands (Orem et al., 2003; Orem et al., 1995).

Paterson and Zderad's humanistic nursing theory

Humanistic nursing practice theory proposes that nurses consciously and deliberately approach nursing as an existential experience. Then, they reflect on the experience and phenomenologically describe the calls they receive, their responses, and what they come to know from their presence in the nursing situation. Humanistic nursing maintains that "nursing is a responsible searching, transactional relationship whose meaningfulness demands conceptualization founded on a nurses existential awareness of self and of the other" (Paterson and Zderad, 2007; Paterson and Zderad, 1976: 7). Existential experience is comprised of uniqueness-otherness, authenticity-experiencing, moreness-choice and value-nonvalue. As noted by Paterson and Zderad (2007), "nurses have the privilege of being with persons who are experiencing all of the varied meanings of incarnate being with men and things in time and space in the entire range from birth to death. They not only have the opportunity to co-experience and co-search with patients the meaning of life, suffering, and death, but in the process they may become and help others become more-more human" (Paterson and Zderad, 1976; Paterson and Zderad, 2007). These tenets respond to palliative care values.

Therefore, Humanistic Nursing Theory is reflected in the World Health Organization's citation of "the need for expert, palliative and end-of-life care as a top priority for global health care" (Wu and Volker, 2012: 471). The theory's philosophical perspectives – moreness-choice; call-and-response; intersubjective transaction; uniqueness-otherness; being and doing and community – are relevant to both hospice and palliative care nursing (Wu and Volker, 2012).

Roy's Adaptation Model

Roy developed the Adaptation Model of Nursing, which depicts the individual as a set of interrelated systems (biological, psychological and social). The individual strives to maintain a balance between and among these systems and the outside world; however, there is no absolute level of balance. Individuals strive to live within a unique band in which he or she can cope adequately. Roy's goal for nursing is promoting adaptation in each of four modes: physiological, self-concept, role function and interdependence. These contribute to the person's health, quality of life and to dying with dignity (Roy, 2009).

Watson's caring science

Watson (2012) identified seven assumptions and ten primary carative factors as the foundation of her theory. The seven assumptions are:

1   Caring can be effectively demonstrated and practiced only interpersonally
2   Caring consists of carative factors that result in the satisfaction of certain human needs
3   Effective caring promotes health and individual or family growth
4   Caring responses accept person not only as he or she is now but as what he or she may become
5   A caring environment is one that offers the development of potential while allowing the person to choose the best action for himself or herself at a given point in time
6   Caring is more "healthogenic" than is curing. A science of caring is complementary to the science of curing
7   The practice of caring is central to nursing.

The four major concepts of her theory are human being, health, environment/society and nursing. The strengths of her theory, which resonate with palliative care nursing, are that it places the client in the context of the family, the community and the culture, and the client is the focus of practice rather than the technology (Watson, 2012).

Parse's Theory of Human Becoming

Parse (1992) changed the name of her theory from "man-living-health" to the Theory of Human Becoming. Her theory arises from the focus on the person as unitary, in mutual process with the environment and on health as a value. Parse focuses on the experience of persons as freely choosing human beings who cocreate health in mutual process with the universe. The person is respected as the expert on his or her own health, and the meaning of lived experience is honored (Parse, 1998; Parse, 1992; Parse, 1995).

Roger's science of unitary human beings

Roger's theory views nursing as both a science and an art. The purpose of nursing is to promote health and well-being in all persons wherever they are. The unitary human being and his or her environment are one. A change of pattern and organization of the human and environmental fields is transmitted by waves. By identifying the pattern, there can be a better understanding of human experience. The eight concepts in Rogers's theory are energy field, openness, pattern, pan-dimensionality, homeodynamic principles, resonance, helicy and integrality (Rogers, 1994).

Middle-range theories of relevance to cancer care

Meleis's theory of transitions

According to Meleis et al. (2000), persons in transition tend to be more vulnerable to risks, which may in turn affect their health. Identifying these risks can be enhanced by understanding the transition process. The theory consists of types and patterns of transitions, properties of transition experiences, facilitating and inhibiting conditions, process indicators, outcome indicators and nursing therapeutics.

McGill model of nursing

The important features of this model are health, family, collaboration and learning within the health, person, environment and nursing paradigm. The goal of this model is "to maintain, strengthen, and develop the patient's health by actively engaging him or her in a learning process" (Gottlieb and Rowat, 1987: 7). This model proposes to focus on the patients and their families. Nurses are essential in the health system to foster the family's health. To achieve this, nurses establish a promoting learning environment. Thus, patient and family participation and subsequent successful learning are supported. In this process, nurses, patients and their families set goals of care together. The patient's strengths and resources are essential elements in the goal setting process. Nurses subsequently employ existing support or develop interventions to promote patient and family health (Gottlieb and Rowat, 1987).

Bandura's social cognitive theory

Bandura addresses the perception of self-competence as influencing the acquisition, development and achievement of competence. The central variable is self-efficacy, which is used interchangeably with competence. Perceived self-competence is defined by social cognitive theory as follows: "People's judgments of their capabilities to organize and execute a course of action requires attaining designated types of performances" (Bandura, 1986: 391). It is believed that nurses with high self-perceived competence demonstrate higher-level care to patients with life-threatening illness and their family. These nurses are more committed to care and persevere in the face of difficulties; quality palliative care requires both nursing competence (acquired and developed through training and experience) and self-competence (Bandura, 1986).

Rodin's attachment theory applied to palliative care

Rodin's attachment theory is a developmentally based approach to our understanding of the formation and maintenance of relationships, which contribute to one's "felt security" (Tan et al., 2005). The core concept of this theory is the attachment that emerges between two persons, be it patient and physician. This theory is relevant to palliative care as the progression of advanced disease presents challenges such as the loss of self-sufficiency to the patient, which results in an increased need for support by others. This increasing reliance on others may activate or reactivate relational problems and may trigger in the patient feelings of vulnerability and dependency. Application of attachment theory in palliative care provides clinicians with guidance in identifying and responding appropriately to the needs of persons receiving end-of-life care (Tan et al., 2005).

Desbiens's palliative care nursing

The authors (Desbiens et al., 2012) describe a new shared theory that combines Bandura's social cognitive theory and Orem's conceptual model, with a focus on the evaluation of nursing education programs in palliative care and the resultant improvement in quality of care and quality of life for patients with life-limiting illness. In this model, the core concepts from Orem's theory, namely self-care agency and self-care as well as the basic conditioning factors are combined with the concept of self-perceived competence from Bandura's social cognitive theory. This new model, which consists of four levels can then be used to determine the needs of palliative care patients (Desbiens et al., 2012).

Reed's theory of self-transference

The key concepts of Reed's Self-Transference theory are: person, environment, health, and nursing. The two major assumptions of the theory are that (a) human beings are integral to their environment and (b) self-transference is a developmental imperative. The major concepts are self-transcendence (intrapersonal, interpersonal, temporal, and transpersonal); well-being; and vulnerability (Reed, 1991). The purpose of this theory is to indicate "developmental phenomena as related to well-being in later life phases" (Reed, 1991: 65). As such, the theory is considered relevant for end of life and palliative care (Reed, 1991).

Theory of unpleasant symptoms

This theory has three major components: the symptoms that the individual is experiencing, the influencing factors that give rise to or affect the nature of the symptom experience, and the consequences of the symptom experience. Lenz et al. (1997: 14) indicate that "symptoms can occur alone or in isolation from one another but that, more often, multiple symptoms are experienced simultaneously. Dyspnoea, for example, is often accompanied by fatigue, and nausea often occurs with pain. Multiple symptoms can occur together as a result of a single event . . . or one symptom can precede another. The concurrence of multiple symptoms is likely to result in an experience that is multiplicative rather than additive". The purpose of this theory is to highlight the interactions between multiple symptoms, to guide symptom management and to subsequently provide tailored interventions to persons suffering from unpleasant symptoms (Lenz et al., 1997).

Symptom management

As noted by Dodd et al. (2001: 669) "a symptom is defined as a subjective experience reflecting changes in the biopsychosocial functioning, sensations, or cognition of an individual. In contrast, a sign is defined as any abnormality indicative of disease that is detectable by the individual or others". In this model, "both signs and symptoms are important cues that bring problems to the attention of patients and clinicians" (Dodd et al., 2001: 669). This model is based on the belief that effective symptom management requires consideration of three dimensions: symptom experience, symptom management strategies and outcomes. Symptom management is a dynamic process; that is, it is modified by individual outcomes and the influences of nursing, domains of person, health/illness or environment.

Theory of uncertainty in illness

While initially focused on persons experiencing the acute phase of illness, the theory now also addresses the experience of living with continual, constant uncertainty in either a chronic disease or in an illness with a treatable acute phase and possible eventual recurrence. Uncertainty is defined by (Mishel, 1990: 256) as "the inability to determine the meaning of illness-related events [which] occurs in situations where the decision-maker is unable to assign definite values to objects and events and/or is unable to accurately predict outcomes because sufficient cues are lacking". The theory's core concept is uncertainty and its appraisal. With this theory, persons suffering from uncertainty are supported by health professionals to think creatively about the ways in which they can continue to have a desired quality of life and to adjust to changes that may occur over time with the trajectory of a chronic illness (Mishel, 1990).

Reed's Unitary-Caring conceptual model for advanced practice nursing in palliative care

Advanced practice nurses contribute to high-quality palliative care. In order to provide a theoretical framework, Reed (2010: 23) proposes a model based on the "unitary-caring approach derived from Rogers' Science of Unitary Human Beings and Watson's Transpersonal Caring Science". The core concepts of this model are "pattern, wholeness, consciousness, caring, transformation and transcendence, relationship, and meaning" (Reed, 2010: 26). The combination of these concepts will guide the advanced practice nurse to provide for palliative care patients.

Murray's transitions model of palliative care

In order to respond to potentially growing palliative care needs, Murray (2007) proposes a model based on the Chronic Condition Management model, which includes palliative care. It is highlighted that the patients' and their families' preferred processes and outcomes are essential to this model. The core concepts of this model are chronic condition management, decision making, palliative care, pattern of care and end of life. Three different patterns of care are identified, namely the patterns of care include "supported self-care, episodic disease management, and case management" (Murray, 2007: 368).

Situation-specific theories

Andershed and Ternestedt's relatives' involvement in the care of the dying

Andershed and Ternestedt (2001) developed a theoretical framework concerning the involvement of families in palliative care based on an in-depth analysis of the outcomes of four earlier studies. An important conclusion they reached was that "the manner in which the staff act toward the patient and relatives influence relatives' possibilities for involvement, patients' possibilities for an appropriate death, and the possibilities the staff have to give good care" (Andershed and Ternestedt, 2001: 554). The core concept of this theory is "meaningful involvement", which consists of an insight, of an enhanced potential from which to choose and of an outcome with impacts on the person or on activities (Andershed and Ternestedt, 2001).

Process of death imminence awareness by family members of patients in adult critical care

In order to better understand the role of family members in relation to persons who require critical care, a grounded theory study was conducted. A substantive middle-range theory emerged with six phases: patient's near-death awareness, dying right in front of me, turning points in the patient's condition, no longer the person I once knew, doing right by them and time to let go. These phases constitute the experience of family members becoming aware that one of their own is dying in critical care (Baumhover, 2015).

Conclusion

While grand theories are referenced in theoretical frameworks applied to cancer, including their influence on middle range theories developed for cancer (e.g., Andershed and Ternestedt (2001), Desbiens et al. (2012), Murray (2007), Reed (1991), Reed (2010)), specific application of theory to cancer has proliferated in the last decade through the emergence of more middle-range theories to guide research, practice and education. Areas of theoretical focus have expanded beyond more specific topics of symptom management and treatment-related issues to address palliative care and overall survivorship. While the largest population of interest involves the patient, increasing focus on palliative care has expanded the population of interest to include family and non-family caregivers to include relationship issues specifically related to cancer treatment, illness trajectories, and survivorship, as well as end-of-life management. Examining emerging conceptual models related to cancer care also highlights the expansion of cancer-related concerns to include more than the physical manifestations or concrete aspects of treatment to include more existential patient and family concerns such as hope, grief and spiritual concerns.

Our systematic review of existing theories highlights the need for further study of the cancer illness trajectory, with focus on social, psychological and spiritual aspects (Murray, 2007). Within this need to address the continuum of patient and family needs throughout survivorship, there is an expanded need to address coping as a dynamic concept in the face of life-threatening (real or perceived) illness (e.g., Mishel (1990), Murray (2007), Shaha (2014)). In addition, it is important to not only address existential concerns at the end of life, but rather view the whole disease trajectory. In an increasingly global society, the impact of cultural bias must be examined in the context of all theories.

Rodin (Tan et al., 2005) has highlighted the importance of relational issues and resulting patient vulnerability and dependency on family or friends. The interface of these relationships with cancer and other health care provider relationships is an important area of focus (Andershed and Ternestedt, 2001). Similarly, the impact of these relationships on each other and the prioritization of key concepts such as empowerment in care negotiations and other patient-family-provider communication should be examined. More recently, Shaha has highlighted that a diagnosis of cancer raises existential issues that influence the disease trajectory. As such, the theory refers to Glaser and Strauss's theory about the disease trajectory of a chronic illness (Glaser and Strauss, 2005), as well as concepts such as uncertainty, locus of control, coping, quality of life and spirituality/existentiality. In addition, a link to Terror Management theory (Harmon-Jones et al., 1997) is suggested. However, further exploration is needed regarding caring, how to navigate patients through the disease trajectory, along with the cultural aspects of the theory.

Specific and focused symptom theories, such as Total Pain Theory, should be linked to existing and related middle-range theories which encompass general symptoms (e.g., Dodd et al. (2001), Lenz et al. (1997), Reed (1991), Reed (2010)). Symptom theories should also be expanded or reviewed to include the relative importance and potential impact of symptom clusters. All symptoms should also be studied in the context of palliative care planning.

In order to effectively address palliative care needs, clear definitions of what palliative care is and what it is not, will become increasingly important (Baumhover, 2015). Theory work, such as that by Desbiens et al. (2012) and Ferrell et al. (2007), highlight the need for further study of ways in which to positively impact nurses' and other health care providers' attitudes about and actions pertaining to palliative care. The End-of-Life Nursing Education Consortium, a national education initiative to improve palliative care, specifically targets oncology providers, along with general geriatric and pediatric populations.

Taken together, in this review, we have identified the need for ongoing theoretical work to directly encompass patient and care partner challenges throughout survivorship. This is especially important given trends related to multimodality treatment, and improved survival, as well as the increasing focus on the long-term sequelae resulting from disease and treatment. Conceptual models of survivorship and liminality are an important move in this direction.

The recognition of cancer disparities and theories which address disparities and social determinants of health will also become increasingly important. As the role of person characteristics and biomarkers of disease expand in the context of precision medicine and as personalized cancer therapies proliferate, there may be and increased role for situation-specific theories or for refinement and revision of existing middle-range theories. As cancer care and treatment advance, the ability to similarly meet the complexities surrounding treatment, symptom management and survivorship issues where multiple theories and concepts intersect may require new ways of developing and applying theory. The rise of interdisciplinary approaches to care and the need to encompass multiple perspectives of the cancer experience may result in the need to develop additional methods to apply and evaluate multiple theories simultaneously.

This systematic approach to reviewing theories in the extant literature has lead us to the following conclusions. There are a few grand theories and some middle-range theories that have been applied in palliative care and oncology settings. While new middle-range theories or conceptual models have and continue to emerge, greater effort must be made to apply these theories and central concepts in a focused manner for future research or for evidence-based practice implementation.

Specific theories carrying the label of "cancer", "oncology", "palliative care" exist in greater scarcity than expected. The question remains: are specific theories needed to guide oncology providers, patients, and families? Although oncology or palliative care patients clearly profit from good social support, few theories or concepts address patients and families. Most of the time, the theories target the patient and nurse/professional-patient relationship.

As leaders in the application of middle range theory to address issues of patient, health, professional practice (i.e., nursing), and environment, nurses are especially well-positioned to advise in the development, implementation and evaluation of theories to guide oncology care of the patient and family. Effective strategies to develop or confirm theory for practice (such as grounded theory) are also part of the nursing research doctorate in the United States and United Kingdom and have been effectively applied in the past. While there is a great theory tradition in the United States and the United Kingdom, theory or concept development elsewhere remains in its infancy. A global approach to middle-range theory development and application will facilitate opportunities to evaluate cultural appropriateness as well as to address the needs of increasingly diverse patient and family populations.

Appendix

Table 3.2 Search of Pubmed/Medline and Cinahl

Database	Search terms	Number of findings	Cited in	Theory	Category
Pubmed/ Medline	("Nursing Theory"[Mesh]) AND ("Palliative Care"[Mesh] OR "Hospice and Palliative Care Nursing"[Mesh] OR "Palliative Medicine"[Mesh])	29	Dobrina et al. (2014) . An overview of hospice and palliative care nursing models and theories.	Desbiens et al. (2012): Shared theory in the field of palliative care nursing based on Bandura's (1986) social cognitive theory and Orem et al.'s (2001) conceptual model.	Middle-range theory
			—	Reed (2010) unitary caring theoretical framework to guide advanced practice nurses based on Watson's transpersonal caring science (Watson and Smith, 2002) and Rogers' science of unitary human beings (Rogers, 1992)	Middle-range theory
			—	Murray (2007) transitions model of palliative care, which aims to integrate palliative nursing services in the context of a chronic condition management model.	Middle-range theory
			Wu and Volker (2012). Humanistic Nursing Theory: application to hospice and palliative care.	Theory to hospice and palliative care nursing based on Paterson and Zderad's publications and other theoretical and research articles and books focused on Humanistic Nursing Theory	Grand theory

(Continued)

Table 3.2 (Continued)

Database	Search terms	Number of findings	Cited in	Theory	Category
			Goebel et al. (2009). Caring for special populations: total pain theory in advanced heart failure: applications to research and practice.	Total pain theory	Concept
			Hutchings (2002). Parallels in practice: palliative nursing practice and Parse's theory of human becoming.	Parse s theory of human becoming and traditional, palliative and hospice nursing practice.	Grand theory
			Penz (2008). Theories of hope: are they relevant for palliative care nurses and their practice?	Concept of hope: Morse and Doberneck (1995), Holtslander et al. (2005), Dufault and Martocchio (1985), Farran et al. (1995)	Concept
			—	Psychological theory of hope based on cognitive psychology by Snyder (1995), Snyder (2002)	Conceptual model
			Andershed and Ternestedt (2001). Development of a theoretical framework describing relatives' involvement in palliative care.	Theoretical framework for relatives' involvement in the care of the dying	Middle-range theory
			Nelson-Marten et al. (1998). Caring theory: a framework for advanced practice nursing.	Watson's theory of caring	Grand theory

Database	Search string	Results	Reference	Concept/theory	Type
Pubmed/Medline	((ethical theory MESH) AND palliative[All Fields]) AND care[All Fields]	21	Braude (2012). Normativity unbound: liminality in palliative care ethics.	Liminality	Concept
Pubmed/Medline	((systems theory MESH) AND ("neoplasms"[MeSH Terms] OR "neoplasms"[All Fields] OR "oncology"[All Fields])) AND care[All Fields]	8	–	–	–
Pubmed/Medline	((psychological theory MESH) AND oncology) AND care	364	Rodin and Zimmermann (2008). Psychoanalytic reflections on mortality: a reconsideration.	Mortality concepts	Concept
Pubmed/Medline	((psychological theory MESH) AND palliative) AND care	160	Tan et al. (2005). Interpersonal processes in palliative care: an attachment perspective on the patient-clinician relationship.	Attachment theory	Middle-range theory
Pubmed/Medline	(((psychological theory MESH) AND oncology) AND palliative) AND care	68	Cutcliffe and Herth (2002). The concept of hope in nursing 1: its origins, background and nature.	Concept of hope	Concept

(Continued)

Table 3.2 (Continued)

Database	Search terms	Number of findings	Cited in	Theory	Category
	((decision theory MESH) AND ("neoplasms"[MeSH Terms] OR "neoplasms"[All Fields] OR "oncology"[All Fields])) AND care[All Fields]	395	–	–	–
	((decision theoryMESH) AND palliative[All Fields]) AND care[All Fields]	74	–	–	–
	((Principle-based ethics MESH) AND oncology) AND care	403	–	–	–
	((Principle-based ethics MESH) AND palliative) AND care	555	–	–	–
	(((Principle-based ethics MESH) AND oncology) AND palliative) AND care	87	Baumrucker et al. (2008). The ethical concept of "best interest".	–	–
	((feminism MESH) AND oncology) AND care	15	–	–	–
	((feminism MESH) AND palliative) AND care	6	–	–	–
	((thanatology MESH) AND ("neoplasms"[All Fields] OR "neoplasms"[MeSH Terms] OR "oncology"[All Fields])) AND care[All Fields]	16	Zimmermann and Rodin (2004). The denial of death thesis: sociological critique and implications for palliative care.	–	–

Search terms	Results	Reference					
((thanatology) AND palliative[All Fields]) AND care[All Fields]	42		—		—		—
((decision making MESH) AND ("neoplasms"[MeSH Terms] OR "neoplasms"[All Fields] OR "oncology"[All Fields])) AND care[All Fields]	3698	Zimmermann and Wennberg (2006). Integrating palliative care: a postmodern perspective.	—				
		—					
((decision making MESH) AND palliative[All Fields]) AND care[All Fields]	2306		—		—		—
(((decision making MESH) AND ("neoplasms"[MeSH Terms] OR "neoplasms"[All Fields] OR "oncology"[All Fields])) AND palliative[All Fields]) AND care[All Fields]							
(((decision making MESH) AND ("neoplasms"[MeSH Terms] OR "neoplasms"[All Fields] OR "oncology"[All Fields])) AND palliative[All Fields]) AND care[All Fields]) AND theory[All Fields]	24	—					—

(Continued)

Table 3.2 (Continued)

Database	Search terms	Number of findings	Cited in	Theory	Category
CINAHL	Major keyword: nursing theory AND major keyword: palliative care	12	Wright and Gros (2012). Theory inspired practice for end-of-life cancer: an exploration of the McGill Model of nursing	McGill Model of Nursing	Middlerange theory
			Mahler (2010). The clinical nurse specialist role in developing a geropalliative model of care.	Watson's Caring-Healing Theory	Grand theory
			McKay et al. (2002). Enhancing palliative care through Watson's carative factors	Watson's Caring-Healing Theory	Grand theory
			Fowler (1994). A welcome focus on a key relationship: using Peplau's model in palliative care	Peplau's model	Grand theory
CINAHL	TX nursing theory AND TX death awareness	3	Baumhover (2015). The Process of Death Imminence Awareness by Family Members of Patients in Adult Critical Care.	Process of Death Imminence Awareness by Family Members of Patients in Adult Critical Care middle-range theory.	Situation-specific theory
CINAHL	Au Ferrell AND tx palliative care	6	Ferrell et al. (2007). The National Agenda for Quality Palliative Care: The National Consensus Project and the National Quality Forum	National Consensus Project for Quality Palliative Care (2009) domains of palliative care.	Conceptual model

Legend: In this table, all MESH-terms that were used to search for the relevant literature, as well as the theories identified are presented, including relevant references.

References

Alligood, M. R. 2013. *Nursing Theorists and their Works*. St. Louis, MO: Mosby/Elsevier.

Andershed, B. and Ternestedt, B. M. 2001. Development of a theoretical framework describing relatives' involvement in palliative care. *Journal of Advanced Nursing*, 34, 554–62.

Bandura, A. 1986. *Social Foundations of Thought and Action: A Social Cognitive Theory*. Englewood Cliffs; London: Prentice-Hall.

Baumhover, N. C. 2015. The process of death imminence awareness by family members of patients in adult critical care. *Dimensions of Critical Care Nursing*, 34, 149–60.

Baumrucker, S. J., Sheldon, J. E., Stolick, M., Morris, G. M., Vandekieft, G. and Harrington, D. 2008. The ethical concept of "best interest". *American Journal of Hospice & Palliative Care*, 25, 56–62.

Braude, H. 2012. Normativity unbound: liminality in palliative care ethics. *Theoretical Medicine and Bioethics*, 33, 107–22.

Cutcliffe, J. R. and Herth, K. 2002. The concept of hope in nursing 1: its origins, background and nature. *British Journal of Nursing*, 11, 832–40.

Cutcliffe, J. R. and McKenna, H. P. 2005. *The Essential Concepts of Nursing: Building Blocks for Practice*. Edinburgh: Elsevier Churchill Livingstone.

Desbiens, J. F., Gagnon, J. and Fillion, L. 2012. Development of a shared theory in palliative care to enhance nursing competence. *Journal of Advanced Nursing*, 68, 2113–24.

Dickoff, J. and James, P. 1968a. Symposium on theory development in nursing. A theory of theories: a position paper. *Nursing Research*, 17, 197–203.

Dickoff, J. and James, P. 1968b. Symposium on theory development in nursing. Researching research's role in theory development. *Nursing Research*, 17, 204–6.

Dobrina, R., Tenze, M. and Palese, A. 2014. An overview of hospice and palliative care nursing models and theories. *International Journal of Palliative Nursing*, 20, 75–81.

Dodd, M., Janson, S., Facione, N., Faucett, J., Froelicher, E. S., Humphreys, J., Lee, K., Miaskowski, C., Puntillo, K., Rankin, S. and Taylor, D. 2001. Advancing the science of symptom management. *Journal of Advanced Nursing*, 33, 668–76.

Dufault, K. and Martocchio, B. C. 1985. Symposium on compassionate care and the dying experience. Hope: its spheres and dimensions. *Nursing Clinics of North America*, 20, 379–91.

Farran, C. J., Herth, K. A. and Popovich, J. M. 1995. *Hope and Hopelessness: Critical Clinical Constructs*. Thousand Oaks, CA; London: Sage.

Fawcett, J. and Desanto-Madeya, S. 2013. *Contemporary Nursing Knowledge: Analysis and Evaluation of Nursing Models and Theories*. Philadelphia, PA: F. A. Davis.

Ferrell, B., Connor, S. R., Cordes, A., Dahlin, C. M., Fine, P. G., Hutton, N., Leenay, M., Lentz, J., Person, J. L., Meier, D. E., Zuroski, K. and National Consensus Project for Quality Palliative Care Task Force, M. 2007. The national agenda for quality palliative care: the National Consensus Project and the National Quality Forum. *Journal of Pain and Symptom Management*, 33, 737–44.

Fowler, J. 1994. A welcome focus on a key relationship. Using Peplau's model in palliative care. *Journal of Professional Nursing*, 10, 194–7.

Glaser, B. G. and Strauss, A. L. 2005. *Awareness of Dying*. New Brunswick, NJ: Aldine Transaction.

Goebel, J. R., Doering, L. V., Lorenz, K. A., Maliski, S. L., Nyamathi, A. M. and Evangelista, L. S. 2009. Caring for special populations: total pain theory in advanced heart failure: applications to research and practice. *Nursing Forum*, 44, 175–85.

Gottlieb, L. and Rowat, K. 1987. The McGill model of nursing: a practice-derived model. *ANS. Advances in Nursing Science*, 9, 51–61.

Harmon-Jones, E., Simon, L., Greenberg, J., Pyszczynski, T., Solomon, S. and McGregor, H. 1997. Terror management theory and self-esteem: evidence that increased self-esteem reduces mortality salience effects. *Journal of Personality and Social Psychology*, 72, 24–36.

Holtslander, L. F., Duggleby, W., Williams, A. M. and Wright, K. E. 2005. The experience of hope for informal caregivers of palliative patients. *Journal of Palliative Care*, 21, 285–91.

Hutchings, D. 2002. Parallels in practice: palliative nursing practice and Parse's theory of human becoming. *American Journal of Hospice & Palliative Medicine*, 19, 408–14.

Im, E. O. 2011. Transitions theory: a trajectory of theoretical development in nursing. *Nursing Outlook*, 59, 278–285 e2.

Lenz, E. R., Pugh, L. C., Milligan, R. A., Gift, A. and Suppe, F. 1997. The middle-range theory of unpleasant symptoms: an update. *ANS. Advances in Nursing Science*, 19, 14–27.

Liehr, P. and Smith, M. J. 1999. Middle range theory: spinning research and practice to create knowledge for the new millennium. *ANS. Advances in Nursing Science*, 21, 81–91.

Mahler, A. 2010. The clinical nurse specialist role in developing a geropalliative model of care. *Clinical Nurse Specialist*, 24, 18–23.

Mcewen, M. and Wills, E. M. 2007. *Theoretical Basis for Nursing*. Philadelphia, PA: Lippincott Williams & Wilkins.

Mckay, P., Rajacich, D. and Rosenbaum, J. 2002. Enhancing palliative care through Watson's carative factors. *Canadian Oncology Nursing Journal*, 12, 34–44.

Meleis, A. I. 2012. *Theoretical Nursing: Development and Progress*. Philadelphia, PA: Wolters Kluwer Health/Lippincott Williams & Wilkins.

Meleis, A. I., Sawyer, L. M., Im, E. O., Hilfinger Messias, D. K. and Schumacher, K. 2000. Experiencing transitions: an emerging middle-range theory. *ANS. Advances in Nursing Science*, 23, 12–28.

Mishel, M. H. 1990. Reconceptualization of the uncertainty in illness theory. *Image – Journal of Nursing Scholarship*, 22, 256–62.

Morse, J. M. and Doberneck, B. 1995. Delineating the concept of hope. *Image – Journal of Nursing Scholarship*, 27, 277–85.

Morse, J. M., Mitcham, C., Hupcey, J. E. and Tason, M. C. 1996. Criteria for concept evaluation. *Journal of Advanced Nursing*, 24, 385–90.

Murray, M. A. 2007. Crossing over: transforming palliative care nursing services for the 21st century. *International Journal of Palliative Nursing*, 13, 366–76.

Nelson-Marten, P., Hecomovich, K. and Pangle, M. 1998. Caring theory: a framework for advanced practice nursing. *Advanced Practice Nursing Quarterly*, 4, 70–7.

Orem, D. E., Renpenning, K. M. and Taylor, S. G. 2003. *Self Care Theory in Nursing: Selected Papers of Dorothea Orem*. New York: Springer Pub.

Orem, D. E., Taylor, S. G. and Renpenning, K. M. 1995. *Nursing: Concepts of Practice*. St. Louis, MO: Mosby.

Orem, D. E., Taylor, S. G. and Renpenning, K. M. 2001. *Nursing: Concepts of Practice*. St. Louis, MO: Mosby.

Parse, R. R. 1992. Human becoming: Parse's theory of nursing. *Nursing Science Quarterly*, 5, 35–42.

Parse, R. R. 1995. *Illuminations: The Human Becoming Theory in Practice and Research*. New York: National League for Nursing Press.

Parse, R. R. 1998. *The Human Becoming School of Thought: A Perspective for Nurses and Other Health Professionals*. Thousand Oaks, CA: Sage.

Paterson, J. G. and Zderad, L. T. 1976. *Humanistic Nursing*. New York: Wiley.

Paterson, J. G. and Zderad, L. T. 2007. *Humanistic Nursing (Meta-Theoretical Essays on Practice)* [Online]. Available at: www.wowcontentclub.com. [Accessed August 2016].

Penz, K. 2008. Theories of hope: are they relevant for palliative care nurses and their practice? *International Journal of Palliative Nursing*, 14, 408–12.

Peterson, S. J. and Bredow, T. S. 2009. *Middle Range Theories: Application to Nursing Research*. Philadelphia, PA: Wolters Kluwer Health/Lippincott Williams & Wilkins.

Reed, P. G. 1991. Toward a nursing theory of self-transcendence: deductive reformulation using developmental theories. *ANS. Advances in Nursing Science*, 13, 64–77.

Reed, S. M. 2010. A unitary-caring conceptual model for advanced practice nursing in palliative care. *Holistic Nursing Practice*, 24, 23–34.

Rodgers, B. L. 2005. *Developing Nursing Knowledge: Philosophical Traditions and Influences*. Philadelphia, PA: Lippincott Williams & Wilkins.

Rodin, G. and Zimmermann, C. 2008. Psychoanalytic reflections on mortality: a reconsideration. *The Journal of the American Academy of Psychoanalysis and Dynamic Psychiatry*, 36, 181–96.

Rogers, M. E. 1992. Nursing science and the space age. *Nursing Science Quarterly*, 5, 27–34.

Rogers, M. E. 1994. The science of unitary human beings: current perspectives. *Nursing Science Quarterly*, 7, 33–5.

Roy, C. 2009. *The Roy Adaptation Model*. Upper Saddle River, NJ: Pearson Prentice Hall.

Roy, C. and Roy Adaptation Association. 2014. *Generating Middle Range Theory: From Evidence to Practice*. New York: Springer Pub.

Shaha, M. 2014. The omnipresence of cancer. In From The Chair of Family Orientated and Community Nursing, F. O. H., Department of Nursing Science (ed.), *Cumulative Thesis in Partial Fulfilment of Obtaining the Venia Legendi for the Subject of Nursing Science of the Faculty of Health, Department of Nursing Science of the University Witten/Herdecke*. Witten/Herdecke, Germany: University of Witten/Herdecke.

Shaha, M. 2016. Die Entwicklung einer MR-Theorie basierend auf phänomenologischer Forschung. *QuPuG*, 15, 15–23.

Smith, M. J. and Liehr, P. R. 2014. *Middle Range Theory for Nursing*. New York, NY: Springer.

Snyder, C. R. 1995. Conceptualizing, measuring, and nurturing hope. *Journal of Counseling & Development*, 73, 355–60.

Snyder, C. R. 2002. Hope theory: rainbows in the mind. *Psychological Inquiry*, 13, 249–75.

Tan, A., Zimmermann, C. and Rodin, G. 2005. Interpersonal processes in palliative care: an attachment perspective on the patient-clinician relationship. *Palliative Medicine*, 19, 143–50.

Watson, J. 2012. *Human Caring Science: A Theory of Nursing*. Sudbury, MA: Jones & Bartlett Learning.

Watson, J. and Smith, M. C. 2002. Caring science and the science of unitary human beings: a trans-theoretical discourse for nursing knowledge development. *Journal of Advanced Nursing*, 37, 452–61.

Wright, D. K. and Gros, C. P. 2012. Theory inspired practice for end-of-life cancer care: an exploration of the McGill Model of Nursing. *Canadian Oncology Nursing Journal*, 22, 175–89.

Wu, H. L. and Volker, D. L. 2012. Humanistic Nursing Theory: application to hospice and palliative care. *Journal of Advanced Nursing*, 68, 471–9.

Zimmermann, C. and Rodin, G. 2004. The denial of death thesis: sociological critique and implications for palliative care. *Palliative Medicine*, 18, 121–8.

Zimmermann, C. and Wennberg, R. 2006. Integrating palliative care: a postmodern perspective. *American Journal of Hospice & Palliative Medicine*, 23, 255–8.

4 Theory of *The Omnipresence of Cancer*

Including two concepts: uncertainty and transitoriness

M. Zumstein-Shaha and C. Cox

Introduction

In this chapter, the theory *The Omnipresence of Cancer* is described. The theory derived its beginning in a qualitative study that employed a phenomenological research design based on Heidegger's Ontology of Dasein[1] (Shaha, 2003a; Shaha and Cox, 2003). Subsequently, to construction of the theory, five studies employing qualitative and quantitative designs have been conducted to further develop and substantiate the theory. In theory building order amongst the five, the first four are: two concept analyses exploring the concepts Uncertainty (Shaha et al., 2008) and Transitoriness (Shaha et al., 2011a), a secondary thematic analysis to further explore the concept of Transitoriness (Shaha and Bauer-Wu, 2009), and a cross-sectional study that explored the associations between the concepts of Uncertainty, Transitoriness, Control and Quality of life (Shaha et al., 2010). This series of studies concluded with an exploration of the contribution of the concept analyses to nursing science (Shaha et al., 2011b). In this chapter, background knowledge associated with cancer will be addressed. Patients' reactions to a diagnosis of cancer and the necessity for developing theory will be presented. A case example that presents the theory, *The Omnipresence of Cancer*, which was derived from research conducted amongst patients with a diagnosis of colorectal cancer follows. The purpose of *The Omnipresence of Cancer*, as a theory, is to facilitate an understanding of having been diagnosed with cancer and its effect on the ontology[2] of human existence multi-dimensionally.

Background

Although the incidence of cancer is declining in first world countries, this disease remains one of the most frequent causes of death in the world. Approximately 13% of all deaths in the world are attributed to cancer (WHO, 2014). The most frequent forms of cancer are located in the breast and the digestive system. The World Health Organisation (WHO) estimates that about 70% of all cancers occur in second and third world (low and middle income) countries. Although research is advancing in relation to cancer treatments, death from cancer is estimated to rise overall to 12 million by the year 2030 (WHO, 2014).

Several causes are perceived as contributing to cancer growth. Some of these causes are external agents such as physical, chemical or biological carcinogens. Age is recognised as an important factor as well as the consumption of alcohol and tobacco. Sedentary lifestyles and a diet high in saturated fat and low in fibre are also considered to be contributing to the development of cancer. Recommendations for reducing the risk of cancer include moderation in the consumption of alcohol, abstinence in the use of tobacco, engagement in moderate exercise and maintaining a healthy diet (WHO, 2014).

Cancer attributes to approximately 45% of lost life-years in women, with breast cancer being the leading cause. In men, cancer accounts for approximately 29% of lost life-years, with prostate cancer being the leading cause (Krebsliga Schweiz, 2012). Although colon and lung cancers have a high incidence and prevalence, many studies focus on breast and prostate cancer patients. There is a need to consider other cancer populations in order to increase an understanding of this disease.

Reactions to a cancer diagnosis – theorising the situation

Research indicates that cancer screening can reveal malignancy (American Cancer Society, 2014). Further testing can reveal the size of a malignant growth and subsequent diagnosis and prognosis that may be communicated to a person. Small and circumscribed cancer sizes indicate more favourable outcomes and higher survival rates than large malignant growths that have already spread throughout a person's body (Siegel et al., 2014). Strict treatment regimens aimed at destroying the malignant growth to ensure disease-free survival often follow a cancer diagnosis. The disease and treatments frequently produce physical side effects and symptoms, such as nausea, vomiting and/or fatigue. A cancer diagnosis, treatments and subsequent side effects impair a person's quality of life and sense of well-being (Institute of Medicine, 2013).

Life after a diagnosis of cancer holds many unknown aspects that constitute challenges patients and significant others must manage. Treatment effects are unknown; the disease trajectory and its influence on everyday life are difficult to foresee, despite information by healthcare providers (Shaha, 2003a; Shaha and Cox, 2003; Ramfelt et al., 2002; Cohen et al., 2004; Mishel et al., 2005; Sarna et al., 2005). Although the extent of the influence of cancer on patients and their significant others is well documented, a theoretical basis for caring has been lacking. Subsequently, helping patients and significant others on how to cope with these challenges is acute.

With confirmation of a cancer diagnosis at the outset of the disease management trajectory, patients experience a sense of life's finitude[3] (Lovgren et al., 2010; Moene et al., 2006; Westman et al., 2006; Cohen et al., 2004; Esbensen et al., 2008). If the aforementioned is addressed early on in the care of cancer patients, a sense of prevention, when a prognosis is good, and preparation for the inevitable, when a prognosis is poor, may be introduced. Patients and significant others may be able to better prepare for the disease trajectory and for an end to life. When a prognosis is poor, with the support of healthcare professionals, patients may eventually be able to experience what is perceived as a good death with dignity. Significant others may gain a better ability to cope and accept death. Further research studies are urgently needed to provide more evidence associated with such issues. In addition, a theory addressing the patients' experience of being diagnosed and living with cancer may assist healthcare professionals to better support patients and significant others during the disease trajectory.

Advances in medical and related sciences, organisational and structural improvements to provide access to state-of-the-art treatments, as well as the institutionalisation of large screening programmes, have contributed to increased success in treatments of cancer. With this, disease-free survival at five years can be obtained for a large number of cancer patients in first world countries. For example, in the United Kingdom, 46% of men and 54% of women diagnosed with cancer survive (Cancer Research UK, 2012), and in the United States, 66.1% of all men and women diagnosed and treated for cancer of all types survive (National Cancer Institute, 2015). Furthermore, in Switzerland, the survival rate of women is 76.2% and for men 69.9% (Sant et al., 2009). In 2010, research found that in countries across Europe, cancer mortality rates were lowest in Cyprus, Finland, Sweden and Switzerland, at under 150 deaths per 100,000 population (OECD iLibrary, 2015).

Despite the fact that a cancer tumour is not growing and therefore does not constitute a health threat, patients still feel in they are in limbo (Shaha and Cox, 2003). A full remission of the disease is considered to be uncertain and unpredictable. Patients are uncertain the cancer will not recur (Frank, 2003; Kenne Sarenmalm et al., 2009; Paterson, 2001). For the majority of cancer patients that have successfully lived through treatments, there is a perceived and potential risk of recurrent disease. Therefore, careful monitoring involving regular consultations occurs throughout the remainder of patients' lives. In many instances, regular monitoring visits to the physician are described by patients as being very stressful (Frank, 2003; Paterson, 2001; Shaha, 2003a; Shaha and Cox, 2003). Hence, for many patients and significant others, survivorship is perceived as limited. Patients and significant others continue to live with the possibility of recurrent disease. Symptoms such as fatigue due to the disease or its treatment also prevail in cancer survivors. Therefore, surviving cancer involves a reordering of a patient's life so that it is adapted to meet the demands of the situation. Not only the cancer survivor is involved, but also their significant others. Assistance may be necessary in order to return to work which research has found is significantly important to cancer survivors (Amir et al., 2008).

Cancer presents as a stigma for many patients which involves a negative connotation (Mosher and Danoff-Berg, 2007; Schulte, 2002; Shaha and Cox, 2003; Westman et al., 2006). The stigma is associated with bodily changes, such as scars from surgical interventions and an inability to maintain previous activities of daily living (Lebel et al., 2007). It also encompasses the sentiment of living in limbo and a constant life-threatening state (Bertero et al., 2008; Kenne Sarenmalm et al., 2009). The sentiment of stigma is an expression of disease related fears and anxiety associated with a threat to life caused by the cancer diagnosis (Mosher and Danoff-Berg, 2007).

In some cases, the spread of the disease cannot be curtailed completely; despite anti-cancer treatments. Metastases and disease progression become manifest (Svensson et al., 2008), thereby increasing feelings of uncertainty and related issues such as finitude of life for patients which subsequently impacts significant others and healthcare professionals (Burnet and Robinson, 2000; Grumann and Spiegel, 2003). Questions arise concerning the outcome of treatments and the influence of the disease on patients' lives and their significant others (Bakitas et al., 2009). Addressing these issues constitutes an important task for healthcare professionals (Mishel and Clayton, 2008; Hagerty et al., 2005). As the experience of uncertainty and transitoriness is an expression of existential upheaval, it is essential that a very basic sense of security is offered, such as listening (McCorkle et al., 2008; Breitbart et al., 2010; Staudacher, 2011). However, additional interventions to support patients and their significant others are in need of development. Therefore, a theoretical basis of the cancer experience is required.

Management of symptoms constitutes a key aspect in the treatment of cancer throughout its disease trajectory. Considerable emphasis is placed on reducing symptom distress due to physical symptoms such as fatigue or pain (Henoch et al., 2008; Heppner et al., 2009; Cleeland, 2007; Currin and Meister, 2008; Manne et al., 2010; Marcus et al., 2010). Psychosocial reactions such as anxiety or uncertainty have been found to play important roles in the disease trajectory of cancer (Barsevick et al., 2006; Bourbonniere and Kagan, 2004; Nelson et al., 2009; Sherman et al., 2010; Sigal et al., 2008). It is therefore essential that psychosocial reactions/behaviours are recognised and treated, as experiencing fewer symptoms contributes to a higher quality of life (Buck et al., 2009; Nelson et al., 2009; Simpson and Whyte, 2006; Julkunen et al., 2009; Thompson et al., 2009).

Disease progression is a difficult and challenging experience. It has been found to be worse than a disease diagnosis, as patients and their significant others already have a detailed knowledge of the disease management that follows

(Kenne Sarenmalm et al., 2009; Svensson et al., 2008). Recurring cancer has also been found to be viewed as a chronic illness (Burnet and Robinson, 2000). For patients, the chronic nature of the illness becomes part of life (Clayton et al., 2008; Curtis et al., 2008; Kenne Sarenmalm et al., 2009). In the "Shifting Perspectives Model of Chronic Illness" (Paterson, 2001; Paterson, 2003), patients are in constant assessment and evaluation of their illness situation in relation to their environment. Their health status and condition is assessed and evaluated in view of their known health status (Paterson, 2001; Paterson, 2003). To some extent, the chronic nature of the disease leads to a new measure and/or a new perspective about the patient's self and health condition. This change in perspective replaces the old view of being healthy (Paterson, 2001; Paterson, 2003). The patient's life may be different than before confirmation of the cancer diagnosis. Re-orientation and re-construction of a patient's life can involve identification and letting go of previously held convictions and beliefs in order to continue living meaningfully (Breitbart, 2002; Harrington et al., 2008; Kenne Sarenmalm et al., 2009; Mehnert et al., 2006; Porter et al., 2009).

Although models such as the "Shifting Perspectives Model of Chronic Illness" (Paterson, 2001; Paterson, 2003; Paterson, 2000) exist, a paucity of studies or theories exist in nursing and healthcare that describe the ontological experience of disease amongst cancer patients. Such paucity prohibits the development and application of caring interventions required to support patients and their significant others during the trajectory of disease management.

Despite many advances in cancer diagnostics and treatment, in improving access to cancer care and establishing screening programmes, cancer ultimately leads to death in many cases. A cancer diagnosis can therefore be perceived as a limiting factor in a person's life (Hubbard et al., 2010; Kenne Sarenmalm et al., 2009; LeMay and Wilson, 2008). Often, cancer patients face a rapid decline at the end-of-life permitting limited time to prepare for death (Lynn and Adamson, 2003). In relation to the end of life in cancer, discussions are needed regarding the place of death (Ahlner-Elmqvist et al., 2004; Burge et al., 2003; Houttekier et al., 2010); adequacy of treatments (Bauvet et al., 2008; Homs et al., 2005); good symptom management (Esper and Heidrich, 2005; Fan et al., 2007; Miaskowski, 2006); institution of palliative care (Homs et al., 2005); involvement of spiritual care (Balboni et al., 2010; Breitbart et al., 2010; Chochinov and Cann, 2005); and support of patients' significant others (Edwards and Clarke, 2004; McMillan et al., 2006; Mellon et al., 2007; Northouse et al., 2010).

In conclusion, the influence of the disease on patients and their significant others is well known and documented. Similarly, the disease trajectory of cancer has been evidenced and described. However, theoretical foundations in nursing and healthcare professions in general are limited which restrains the development of new roles and activities. Furthermore, the development and evaluation of adequate interventions are limited. Research is required that provides a basis for theory development and implementation associated with nursing's and healthcare professionals' role in the management of patients diagnosed with cancer.

Discussion

Development of theory

As presented in the introduction to this chapter, in relation to the aforementioned, a series of studies were conceptualised and conducted to discern a nursing theory (which can be applicable to other healthcare professions) about being diagnosed and living with cancer. Initially, a qualitative study using a phenomenological design, drawing on Heidegger's Ontology of Dasein[1], was conducted (Shaha, 2003a; Shaha and Cox, 2003; Shaha et al., 2006). A series of interviews were undertaken with seven patients (four men, mean age 64.5 years; three women, mean age 67 years; age range 49–80 years). The interviews were transcribed and analysed using Colaizzi's analytic steps as described in Haase (Haase, 1987: 66–67). One main category and two subcategories were identified. These were *The Omnipresence of Cancer*, Toward Authentic Dasein and Mapping Out the Future. Being diagnosed and living with cancer is described as an overwhelming experience influencing the totality of an individual. Cancer becomes the primary focus of an individual's life and is seen as being omnipresent. Treatments dictate the daily structure of life. After completion of treatments, regular monitoring shapes an individual's life. In the presence of a cancer diagnosis, a number of questions arise. Individuals ask about the reasons and causes for the disease. They are uncertain about their future and they recognise the finitude[3] of their life. It is probable that some individuals delegate decisions to other people, such as the healthcare professionals, because they have an inability to cope with their situation. Questioning offers an opportunity to gain a glimpse of themselves, which can enrich life. However, the disease remains a constant reminder in an individuals' life. Therefore, the individual has to find a way to accept the disease and its probable outcome. Once again, an individual is confronted with many questions regarding daily life including work. They are uncertain about the influence of the illness on daily life and the future. As time evolves, individuals affected by a cancer diagnosis and treatment may reflect on the influence the finitude of life has and revoke delegation of decisions to others and assume control of their healthcare management.

The qualitative phenomenological study provided the foundation for discernment of the theory *The Omnipresence of Cancer* with its sub-categories Toward Authentic Dasein' and Mapping Out the Future. Within the sub-categories, three concepts were identified, namely Uncertainty, Transitoriness and Control.

Although the foundation of the theory was discerned and constructed, further research was considered necessary in order to develop a middle range theory. Two concept analyses were conducted. The first aimed at describing the concept of Uncertainty. For this concept analysis, a comprehensive literature review was undertaken in order to generate concept clarification (Shaha et al., 2008). Three main aspects of uncertainty were revealed. It was found that adequate information about the disease, its associated treatments, side effects and illness trajectory are seen as contributing to the underlying characteristics of uncertainty. In addition, an existential aspect of uncertainty was revealed. Patients and their significant others experience uncertainty in relation to their life and coping (Shaha et al., 2008). Therefore, information should be tailored to patients' and their significant others' needs and provided in a comprehensive fashion that promotes acceptance and coping with the disease (Shaha et al., 2008).

The second concept analysis focused on transitoriness. An evolutionary concept analysis was employed to develop this concept. Three main characteristics were identified. The experience of transitoriness means that patients become aware of the finitude of their lives. Confrontation with finitude of life provokes anxiety. However, changes can become possible because of this realisation (Shaha et al., 2011a). Subsequently, a secondary qualitative thematic analysis was conducted to further explore the concept of transitoriness, which was part of a larger randomised controlled study to determine the effect of expressive writing on the coping of young women with breast cancer. The texts written as part of the expressive writing assignment were compiled and underwent thematic analysis. Three main themes emerged. Women wrote about their thoughts of being remembered by their significant others. In the texts, women described a landscape of emotions and perspectives. They wrote about the omnipresence of cancer and its influencing effect on life's finitude (Shaha and Bauer-Wu, 2009).

As part of a quantitative cross-sectional study among patients with aerodigestive tract cancers the relationships between uncertainty, elements of transitoriness, control, and quality of life were explored. Significant associations were determined between these variables. The more uncertainty, transitoriness, or belief in chance individuals experience, the lower their quality of life. Finally, the contribution of concept analysis to theory building in nursing was explored. A retroductive study design was employed, including a comprehensive literature review on theory building and concept analysis. Findings demonstrated that in nursing, concept analysis is controversial. However, concepts are acknowledged as building blocks of theories and therefore indispensable in theory development. The development and description of concepts contributes to clarification of theories. Depending on the level of concretisation of concepts, theory range can be determined. Abstract and broad concepts are more indicative of grand theories; whereas more concrete, fully described concepts are often part of middle range theories (Shaha et al., 2011b). Based on all of the research and employing a ret-roductive design, the theory *The Omnipresence of Cancer* has emerged at middle range theory level with two partial practice theories emerging. These are Uncertainty and Transitoriness.

The Omnipresence of Cancer

The aim of *The Omnipresence of Cancer* is to provide a description of the experience of being diagnosed with and living with cancer. Based on its description, explanation and prediction, adequate coping strategies and supportive interventions can be developed and proposed to deal with the demands of the illness and its trajectory.

The theory's main category, *The Omnipresence of Cancer*, encompasses the experience of living with cancer. Being diagnosed with cancer constitutes an existential upheaval and signifies a thorough change in the familiar circumstances of life. Invasive and intensive treatments and tight treatment schedules dictate everyday life. As stated previously, the disease consumes everyday life. In addition, even after successful completion of treatments, patients have to undergo regular monitoring for the remainder of their lives (Moene et al., 2006; Steel et al., 2008; Molassiotis et al., 2010). Cancer encroaches on patients' lives, and becomes an omnipresent element of daily life. *The Omnipresence of Cancer* constitutes the outcome of the experience of living with cancer. It addresses changed values and priorities in life, having thoughts about the disease, particularly in relation to health problems such as infection and being concerned about the disease's progression. These are amplified when undergoing regular monitoring.

Measurement of the theory, *The Omnipresence of Cancer*, is important for the future of cancer care. Due to medical progress cancer has been relegated to being considered a chronic illness for many patients (e.g., men living with prostate cancer and patients with multiple myeloma). Regular monitoring of the disease constitutes a source of anxiety and stress. Treatments are frequently provided in outpatient settings, which provides excellent opportunities for patient and family education that can emerge into well organised self-management of the condition. Furthermore, regular medical and nursing consultations can be provided, which are an indispensable part of the cancer trajectory (Ferrell et al., 2013; Paton et al., 2013; Weaver et al., 2013). With these provisions in mind, understanding the experience of *The Omnipresence of Cancer* is important for theory development that determines the kind and time point of suitable interventions to support patients and their significant others.

Toward Authentic Dasein and Mapping Out the Future

The two dimensions Towards Authentic Dasein and Mapping Out the Future underpin the main category (theme) *The Omnipresence of Cancer*. These two dimensions (sub-categories) reflect temporal aspects in the cancer trajectory and living with cancer over time.

Towards Authentic Dasein refers to an early part in the cancer trajectory. It involves the confirmation of the diagnosis, the breaking of 'bad news' and in some cases early surgical intervention. Patients who find themselves in this dimension are thrown back onto themselves. They raise questions about the cause of the disease and/or life with the disease. Obtaining adequate information about the disease and the illness trajectory is essential. Patients' psychosocial reactions demand empathy and empathetic listening (an open ear) (Shaha and Cox, 2003; Birnie et al., 2010; Mehnert, 2006). Patients need to be able to attribute meaning to their experiences in order to make sense of them and to adjust life to the new situation (Lebel et al., 2007; Duggleby et al., 2010).

The dimension of Towards Authentic Dasein comprises three concepts. These are: Uncertainty, Transitoriness and Control. At the outset of the disease, patients are uncertain about the treatment success and the subsequent development of the disease. They are uncertain about their recovery and their return to daily life. An important way to deal with these uncertainties is access to and the provision of tailored information that patients and their significant others can utilise. Information often targets illness specific aspects and less often existential issues that cancer patients also experience (Shaha et al., 2008). To date, one validated and reliable instrument exists that allows for the comprehensive assessment of individual levels of uncertainty (Mishel, 1981). This instrument, however, focuses on the lack of illness related information, is elaborate and has predominantly been used in research. An assessment instrument of uncertainty for practice is therefore important and in need of development. Supporting cancer patients in their experience of uncertainty needs to include re-assessment of the actual situation and a re-formulation of life's goals (McCorkle et al., 2009; Bertero et al., 2008; Bennett et al., 2007). Interventions combining symptom management and self-care reduce uncertainty and contribute to a better quality of life (Gil et al., 2006; Wonghongkul et al., 2006). Adequate interventions addressing the existential aspects of uncertainty need yet to be developed so that patients are better supported in their disease management.

Transitoriness is another concept which is part of the dimension of *Towards Authentic Dasein*. Cancer, in many respects, remains a fatal and life-limiting disease. Therefore, the confirmation of a cancer diagnosis provokes confrontation with life's finitude.[3] The subsequent treatment regimen can also give rise to questions about the finitude of life. Facing life's transitory nature can provoke anxiety and fear and thoughts of death. It can also contribute to a critical review of a person's beliefs, values and priorities.

Assessing the experience of Transitoriness is limited, to date.[4] It is possible to use measures of death anxiety such as the Collett-Lester Fear of Death Scale, or the Templer's Death Anxiety Scale (Robinson and Wood, 1983). A scale that measures the perception of approaching death has also been developed (Vollmer et al., 2011). However, these scales are predominantly psychological in nature and used in research. They are not practical for everyday use by healthcare professionals to ascertain a patient's level of concern regarding the transitory nature of life or associated care requisites.

In psychology and nursing, similar concepts such as fear of death (Penson et al., 2005) or death anxiety (Bassett, 2007) have been developed and included in theories such as 'Terror Management Theory' (Taubman-Ben-Ari et al., 2002). This theory maintains that life-threatening large scale events, such as terrorist attacks, provoke awareness of life's transitory nature in the targeted population. By reinforcing social and personal relationships the population strives to rebuild confidence and trust. Interventions fostering the re-building of or strengthening relationships between individuals or art-based interventions such as painting and drawing have been shown to be supportive. Employment of these interventions shows that individuals feel better able to manage their lives (Mikulincer et al., 2003; Arndt et al., 2005).

Finally, control has been identified as a concept within the dimension of Toward Authentic Dasein. With the diagnosis of cancer and the subsequent treatment regimen, patients have to make decisions regarding their health and treatment. At this period in time, patients rely on health professionals' recommendations. Patients frequently delegate some decisions to healthcare professionals due to their professional competence and knowledge. However, over time, patients often resume control of decision making in order to maintain control of their lives. The concept of control as part of *The Omnipresence of Cancer* is in need of full delineation.

To date, there exist some scales that measure locus of control such as the Health-Related Locus of Control scale by Wallston (2005) and the Rotter Locus of Control scale (Citrin et al., 2012). However, these scales are discussed controversially as the concept itself requires further clarification. Development of an instrument that can adequately measure a patient's level of control would be an essential addition to the concepts inherent in *The Omnipresence of Cancer.* In conclusion, few interventions target control; among these are activity motivating interventions (Rogers et al., 2011) and empowering interventions through self-help groups (Stang and Mittelmark, 2010). Nevertheless, further exploration of supportive interventions targeting control as described in *The Omnipresence of Cancer* is needed.

Mapping Out the Future follows the dimension of Toward Authentic Dasein. Mapping Out the Future indicates the patients' preoccupation with daily life, the influence of the disease on daily life and efforts made by patients and significant others in developing suitable coping strategies to deal with the challenges of the disease situation. Patients bring with them a range of coping strategies and select from among these those that appear most appropriate or helpful to them. Therefore, selecting and employing coping strategies is a highly individualised process. It depends on the coping strategies available to people and their associated experiences. There is evidence that optimism, a fighting spirit and hope are often used as coping strategies by cancer patients and their significant others (Chochinov et al., 2006; Clayton et al., 2005; Northouse et al., 2007). By contrast, anger, avoidance and denial are considered less fruitful coping strategies but are also employed by cancer patients (Aarstad et al., 2008; Julkunen et al., 2009; Timmermans et al., 2007).

In review, patients and their significant others continue to experience uncertainty throughout the illness trajectory (Frenkel et al., 2010; Grimsbo et al., 2011). Patients cannot be sure that the disease is eliminated and will not recur. The remainder of patients' lives is governed by constant vigilance (Geiger et al., 2006; Andrykowski et al., 2008). Depending on the disease stage, progression can be likely. In these situations, patients face, once again, their uncertainties concerning the development of the disease trajectory, and the influence of the disease on daily life. Determining the levels of uncertainty, including the differentiation between information needs and the more existential aspects, is key to providing specific support and care to patients.

When cancer becomes a life-limiting illness, patients continue to experience transitoriness. Their anxiety and fear remain as well as thoughts about death. In order to manage this experience, some patients consider the end of their life and initiate funeral preparations. The experience of transitoriness can lead patients to reconsider their lives, to develop new priorities and/or to change their life-styles (Shaha et al., 2011a; Shaha et al., 2011b; Shaha et al., 2006; Shaha et al., 2010). Patients experience profound changes in their outlook on life. This influences the relationships cancer patients have with their significant others and other important aspects of their lives (McCorry et al., 2009; Sanatani et al., 2008; McMillan et al., 2006). Evaluating the experience of transitoriness regularly throughout the cancer trajectory contributes to providing tailored information and support to patients and their significant others.

In consideration of daily life and finding ways to cope with the demands of the illness, patients reconsider delegation of decision making to health professionals. Patients often resume control over their decisions that had previously been relinquished (Shaha, 2003a; Shaha and Cox, 2003; Shaha et al., 2006). In relation to building middle-range theory, further exploration of these aspects is necessary. Such knowledge will contribute to the development of practice theory that provides individualised interventions and support to patients and their significant others.

Cancer as a disease, with all of its dimensions, concerns patients' significant others, influences daily life and existing relationships. The world of anti-cancer treatments is new to most significant others and few support structures exist to support significant others (Gilbar and Zusman, 2007; Khalili, 2007). Couples, in particular, need to find ways to adjust to the situation (Northouse, 2005; Northouse et al., 2010). There is a danger that relationships can disintegrate in face of the challenges of the disease (Harden, 2005; Esbensen et al., 2008).

Theories address phenomena that are specific as well as abstract in scope (Fawcett, 2005). Grand theories are abstract and broad in scope. As described in Chapter 1 of this book, in grand theory, concepts and are abstract and general. However, at the middle-range theory level, concepts and propositions are more specific. In the narrative that follows, Table 4.1 demonstrates the constructs within the theory *The Omnipresence of Cancer* and its propositions.

Within the theory, the following propositions are identified:

- *The Omnipresence of Cancer* constitutes the outcome of the reactions and the experience of being diagnosed with cancer.
- *The Omnipresence of Cancer* is the result of a high positive association between uncertainty, transitoriness and locus of control.
- *The Omnipresence of Cancer* results in a moderate to low level of quality of life and well-being in cancer patients.
- *The Omnipresence of Cancer* involves active coping.
- *The Omnipresence of Cancer* accounts for changes in life priorities and lifestyle.

Table 4.1 Model of *The Omnipresence of Cancer*

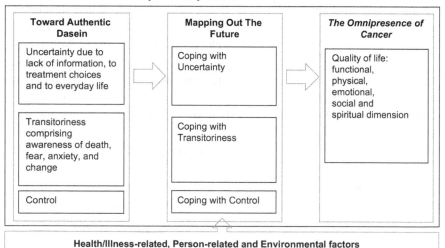

Legend: *The Omnipresence of Cancer* constitutes the outcome variable in this model. It includes quality of life. The dimension of Toward Authentic Dasein encompasses Uncertainty, Transitoriness and Control. Similarly, the dimension of Mapping Out the Future also encompasses Uncertainty, Transitoriness and Control, but specifically in relation to coping.

- *The Omnipresence of Cancer* reduces families' quality of life and well-being.
- Towards Authentic Dasein encompasses differing levels of uncertainty, transitoriness and a change from an internal locus of control to an external locus of control in newly diagnosed cancer patients.
- Mapping Out the Future encompasses differing levels of uncertainty, transitoriness and a change from an external to internal locus of control in newly diagnosed cancer patients.
- Towards Authentic Dasein provokes uncertainty, changes in relationships and distress in families.
- Mapping Out the Future provokes changes in relationships and distress in families.

Case example for practice

The case presented here represents interview and diary narrative from a 50-year-old female German-speaking cancer patient. Narrative substantiates the main category and sub-categories present in *The Omnipresence of Cancer.*

Day 1

Oh Gott, the vomiting won't stop. My insides are spilling out of my mouth. The taste is foul and this Furcht und Angst are all consuming. It is unglaublich! The vomiting won't stop . . . won't stop. Oh Gott, help me . . . help me. Warum ich? Warum ich?

Day 5

It has been there, growing silently. I've known it. They say they don't know if they have gotten it all. So I wait and wait. There is so much waiting and loneliness. The uncertainty is driving me mad! Darmkrebs they say . . . its Darmkrebs. The thoughts won't go away . . . I don't know what to do anymore. There is no way out. I'll leave it to them to decide.

Day 26

I'm dying . . . Yes it is probably so. I've seen my face. I can't look at it any more. The lines . . . I've lost my hair. I am no longer the same. The ugly growth that they cut from me is on the outside now. It shows in my eyes, my skin and the bag on my belly . . . it is foul . . . foul. It is the Chemotherapie und Darmkrebs . . . they are killing me!

Day 30

Darmkrebs, oh Gott. Where did it come from? How did I get it? I have always been careful about what I eat. I don't drink and smoke. This is unglaublich! My Furcht und Angst are overwhelming, my emotions are running out of control. My thoughts won't let me rest. Nothing is in my control. Nothing is like it was before. Everything has changed . . . since the diagnosis. Warum ich? Warum ich?

Day 33

Where is my future? I can't imagine any kind of future . . . not anymore. What about the trip my husband and I were going to take next year? If I live, will I be able to travel at all? How will it be? Will he want me with this scar on my belly and this bag? How can he stand to look at me now? I can't stand to look at myself. I'm ugly . . . this thing is hideous! I might be dead in a year. What does it matter now? Warum ich? Warum ich? Why does this thing stay with me? Always there. What have I done wrong?

Day 36

The doctors and nurses are trying to be supportive, despite their lack of time. This hospital is a foul place. It smells of death. It smells like me. I wait. I am alone. Warten und Einsamkeit. I must be dying . . . the smell of death, the rot and decay, they are all around me. Warten und Einsamkeit. The thoughts of it are in my mind. It is like a broken record, playing over and over again. Everything is so uncertain. There is no escape.

Day 37

The doctors and nurses are talking about me going home. I don't know how this will work out. Everything is so uncertain now. There is the colostomy . . . Will I ever live a normal life again? My life has been taken over by the Krebs. I can't plan ahead. Others make decisions for me. In some ways, this has been a relief.

Day 60

I have changed. The Chemotherapie is over. I've stopped it. I couldn't stand the treatment on a daily basis with continuous nausea and vomiting. My insides have rotted away . . . the foul smell. It is always there. I can't keep any nourishment down, however much I try. Even the advice doctors and nurses give does not help.

Table 4.2 Translation

Oh Gott = Oh God
Furcht und Angst = Fear and Anxiety
Unglaublich = Unbelieveable
Warum ich? = Why me?
Darmkrebs = Colorectal Cancer
Chemotherapie = Chemotherapy
Warten und Einsamkeit = I can't escape my thoughts.
So kann es nicht weitergehen = I cannot go on like this.
Krebs = Cancer

Legend: *The Omnipresence of Cancer*, Doctoral Thesis, City
University London (M. Shaha, 2003a)

So kann es nicht weitergehen. I know my decision will have grave implications.
But, I do not want to be miserable until I die. I want to live fully and enjoy what
time I have left. I must take control of what time remains.

Six months later

Since the Chemotherapie was stopped I have felt better. That was six months ago.
The two screenings I've had have been good. The screenings are a terrible ordeal.
Each time I dread the outcome. Furcht und Angst . . . It is all consuming. Everything is uncertain. Will I be able to make my own decisions up until the end? Life
has changed. Everywhere I look, Krebs is there. Nothing is like it used to be. It is
everywhere. It is always with me.

In order to accompany this patient throughout her disease trajectory, a comprehensive assessment of symptoms, level of uncertainty, transitoriness and control
is necessary at regular intervals. A patient such as the patient presented in the Case
Example for Practice will need information regarding the disease, development of
the disease, treatment modalities and associated symptoms (Bertero et al., 2008).
It will be important to provide tailored education so as to empower the patient to
manage the illness. Offering an open ear, discussing the illness experience with
the patient and identifying issues concerning thoughts of death will be important (Balboni et al., 2010; Staudacher, 2011). Based on coping strategies already
mobilised by the patient, interventions such as mindfulness-based stress reduction (Ledesma and Kumano, 2009) can be offered. It will be important to include
significant others in all these activities in order to promote an adaptation to a life
in which cancer is or has been present. Determining attainable goals together with
the patient and her significant others involving telephone follow-ups following
discharge from hospital that address symptoms is essential. In addition providing
education in calming techniques such as breathing techniques can be supportive
(Mishel et al., 2005; Gil et al., 2006). In some cases, calming relaxation techniques

based on imaging can be included with breathing techniques (Lauver et al., 2007; McCorkle et al., 2009; McMillan et al., 2006). *The Omnipresence of Cancer*, as a middle-range theory, can be of assistance in developing and evaluating adequate interventions. Successful management of cancer, however, needs to include all individuals involved in the situation; not just the patient. Therefore, a multi-disciplinary team approach should be called upon to determine together with patients and families the most appropriate interventions for providing support.

Conclusion

Future developments

The Omnipresence of Cancer focuses on cancer patients and their significant others. As the theory is based on the experiences of cancer patients, health in this theory is related to cancer and its implications. However, it is evident that in relation to Toward Authentic Dasein and Mapping Out the Future, there are salient elements that can relate to all aspects of diseases requiring care in Long Term Conditions and Palliative Care. In particular, more detail is required to explicate practice theory in nursing and nurses' roles. In consideration of extension of the theory into the care and management of Long Term Conditions and Palliative Care, further exploration of this theory is essential in order to explore its descriptive, explanatory and predictive powers.

Future research should include the two dimensions Toward Authentic Dasein and Mapping Out the Future in order to determine their interrelationship with time. To develop adequate interventions, the different levels of uncertainty across an illness trajectory, and the experience of transitoriness need to be explored along with the concept of control. It is important to determine the best time points at which tailored interventions can be provided to patients and their significant others so that they can cope better with challenges associated with the illness situation. Measurement instruments of the two dimensions, and each concept and proposition within *The Omnipresence of Cancer*, must be developed for the benefit of patients and their significant others.

For example, new ways of managing cancer, as a disease, on a daily basis need to be developed for patients and significant others. Healthcare professionals must have access to the latest evidence about the disease and its treatments, and be educated to provide support to patients and their significant others. Nursing and other treatment standards need to be evidence-based and accessible to all professionals caring for cancer patients and their significant others (Adams and Titler, 2010).

New models of care that integrate a collaborative and interdisciplinary approach need to be implemented and evaluated (Martin et al., 2010). Among these models the role of the Advanced Practice Nurse (Advanced Nurse Practitioner) constitutes important progress in nursing practice. Advanced Practice Nurses support the integration of new and innovative knowledge, the implementation of tailored interventions, the promotion of nursing at the bedside, the fostering of interdisciplinary collaboration and an ethically sensitive attitude (Hamric et al., 2014). Follow-up visits during and after conclusion of anti-cancer treatments support patients' and significant others' coping processes and re-adaptation and modification of life-style (Badger et al., 2005; McCorkle et al., 2009; Northouse et al., 2010). Advanced Practice Nurses have adopted the role of engaging in such visits. It is time for new models that address disciplines outside of Advanced Practice Nursing to come to the fore.

Being diagnosed and living with cancer is a complex experience influencing all aspects of patients' and their significant others' lives. Patients experience an existential questioning of their lives and meaning of life. Good relationships with patients and their significant others are essential to support them in overcoming the demands of the disease situation and how they are influenced by the disease. At present, nursing roles and the roles of other healthcare professions in relation to interventions are only partially delineated.

The middle-range nursing theory of *The Omnipresence of Cancer* provides a description of the experience of being diagnosed and living with cancer. Thus, the situation of patients and their significant others can be better understood. By employing this middle-range theory, nurses are better able to identify areas for and to plan adequate interventions tailored to the needs of patients and their significant others. Formulating *The Omnipresence of Cancer* as an outcome, healthcare professionals have a means to understand the burden of the disease on patients and their significant others. Thus, monitoring of *The Omnipresence of Cancer* will help in the identification of crisis situations.

Notes

1 Dasein is a German word that means 'being there' or 'presence'.
2 Ontology means specification of a conceptualisation.
3 Finitude means a state of having limits or bounds (e.g., the end of life).
4 An instrument to assess Transitoriness is discussed in Chapter 7.

References

Aarstad, A. K., Aarstad, H. J. and Olofsson, J. 2008. Personality and choice of coping predict quality of life in head and neck cancer patients during follow-up. *Acta Oncologica*, 47, 879–90.

Adams, S. and Titler, M. G. 2010. Building a learning collaborative. *Worldviews on Evidence-Based Nursing*, 7, 165–73.

Ahlner-Elmqvist, M., Jordhoy, M. S., Jannert, M., Fayers, P. and Kaasa, S. 2004. Place of death: hospital-based advanced home care versus conventional care. A prospective study in palliative cancer care. *Palliative Medicine*, 18, 585–93.

American Cancer Society. 2014. *American Cancer Society Guidelines for the Early Detection of Cancer*, ed. by American Cancer Society. Atlanta: American Cancer Society.

Amir, Z., Neary, D. and Luker, K. 2008. Cancer survivors' views of work 3 years post diagnosis: a UK perspective. *European Journal of Oncology Nursing*, 12, 190–7.

Andrykowski, M. A., Lykins, E. and Floyd, A. 2008. Psychological health in cancer survivors. *Seminars in Oncology Nursing*, 24, 193–201.

Arndt, J., Routledge, C., Greenberg, J. and Sheldon, K. M. 2005. Illuminating the dark side of creative expression: assimilation needs and the consequences of creative action following mortality salience. *Personality & Social Psychology Bulletin*, 31, 1327–39.

Badger, T., Segrin, C., Meek, P., Lopez, A. M., Bonham, E. and Sieger, A. 2005. Telephone interpersonal counseling with women with breast cancer: symptom management and quality of life. *Oncology Nursing Forum*, 32, 273–9.

Bakitas, M., Lyons, K. D., Hegel, M. T., Balan, S., Brokaw, F. C., Seville, J., Hull, J. G., Li, Z., Tosteson, T. D., Byock, I. R. and Ahles, T. A. 2009. Effects of a palliative care intervention on clinical outcomes in patients with advanced cancer: the Project ENABLE II randomized controlled trial. *Journal of the American Medical Association*, 302, 741–9.

Balboni, T. A., Paulk, M. E., Balboni, M. J., Phelps, A. C., Loggers, E. T., Wright, A. A., Block, S. D., Lewis, E. F., Peteet, J. R. and Prigerson, H. G. 2010. Provision of spiritual care to patients with advanced cancer: associations with medical care and quality of life near death. *Journal of Clinical Oncology*, 28, 445–52.

Barsevick, A. M., Dudley, W. N. and Beck, S. L. 2006. Cancer-related fatigue, depressive symptoms, and functional status: a mediation model. *Nursing Research*, 55, 366–72.

Bassett, J. F. 2007. Psychological defenses against death anxiety: integrating Terror Management Theory and Firestone's Separation Theory. *Death Studies*, 31, 727–50.

Bauvet, F., Klastersky, J. and Awada, A. 2008. Supportive care in cancer: concepts, achievements and challenges. *Bulletin du Cancer*, 95, 381–8.

Bennett, P., Phelps, C., Brain, K., Hood, K. and Gray, J. 2007. A randomized controlled trial of a brief self-help coping intervention designed to reduce distress when awaiting genetic risk information. *Journal of Psychosomatic Research*, 63, 59–64.

Bertero, C., Vanhanen, M. and Appelin, G. 2008. Receiving a diagnosis of inoperable lung cancer: patients' perspectives of how it affects their life situation and quality of life. *Acta Oncologica*, 47, 862–9.

Birnie, K., Garland, S. N. and Carlson, L. E. 2010. Psychological benefits for cancer patients and their partners participating in mindfulness-based stress reduction (MBSR). *Psycho-Oncology*, 19, 1004–9.

Bourbonniere, M. and Kagan, S. H. 2004. Nursing intervention and older adults who have cancer: specific science and evidence based practice. *Nursing Clinics of North America*, 39, 529–43.

Breitbart, W. 2002. Spirituality and meaning in supportive care: spirituality- and meaning-centered group psychotherapy interventions in advanced cancer. *Supportive Care in Cancer*, 10, 272–80.

Breitbart, W., Rosenfeld, B., Gibson, C., Pessin, H., Poppito, S., Nelson, C., Tomarken, A., Timm, A. K., Berg, A., Jacobson, C., Sorger, B., Abbey, J. and Olden, M. 2010. Meaning-centered group psychotherapy for patients with advanced cancer: a pilot randomized controlled trial. *Psycho-Oncology*, 19, 21–8.

Buck, H. G., Overcash, J. and McMillan, S. C. 2009. The geriatric cancer experience at the end of life: testing an adapted model. *Oncology Nursing Forum*, 36, 664–73.

Burge, F., Lawson, B. and Johnston, G. 2003. Trends in the place of death of cancer patients, 1992–1997. *Canadian Medical Association Journal*, 168, 265–70.

Burnet, K. and Robinson, L. 2000. Psychosocial impact of recurrent cancer. *European Journal of Oncology Nursing*, 4, 29–38.

Cancer Research UK. 2012. *Cancer Statistics*. London: Cancer Research UK.

Chochinov, H. M. and Cann, B. J. 2005. Interventions to enhance the spiritual aspects of dying. *Journal of Palliative Medicine*, 8(Suppl 1), S103–15.

Chochinov, H. M., Kristjanson, L. J., Hack, T. F., Hassard, T., McClement, S. and Harlos, M. 2006. Personality, neuroticism, and coping towards the end of life. *Journal of Pain & Symptom Management*, 32, 332–41.

Citrin, D. L., Bloom, D. L., Grutsch, J. F., Mortensen, S. J. and Lis, C. G. 2012. Beliefs and perceptions of women with newly diagnosed breast cancer who refused conventional treatment in favor of alternative therapies. *Oncologist*, 17, 607–12.

Clayton, J. M., Butow, P. N., Arnold, R. M. and Tattersall, M. H. 2005. Fostering coping and nurturing hope when discussing the future with terminally ill cancer patients and their caregivers. *Cancer*, 103, 1965–75.

Clayton, M. F., Dudley, W. N. and Musters, A. 2008. Communication with breast cancer survivors. *Health Communication*, 23, 207–21.

Cleeland, C. S. 2007. Symptom burden: multiple symptoms and their impact as patient-reported outcomes. *Journal of the National Cancer Institutes Monographs*, 16–21.

Cohen, M. Z., Williams, L., Knight, P., Snider, J., Hanzik, K. and Fisch, M. J. 2004. Symptom masquerade: understanding the meaning of symptoms. *Supportive Care in Cancer*, 12, 184–90.

Currin, J. and Meister, E. A. 2008. A hospital-based intervention using massage to reduce distress among oncology patients. *Cancer Nursing*, 31, 214–21.

Curtis, J. R., Engelberg, R., Young, J. P., Vig, L. K., Reinke, L. F., Wenrich, M. D., McGrath, B., McCown, E. and Back, A. L. 2008. An approach to understanding the interaction of hope and desire for explicit prognostic information among individuals with severe chronic obstructive pulmonary disease or advanced cancer. *Journal of Palliative Medicine*, 11, 610–20.

Duggleby, W., Holtslander, L., Steeves, M., Duggleby-Wenzel, S. and Cunningham, S. 2010. Discursive meaning of hope for older persons with advanced cancer and their caregivers. *Canadian Journal on Aging*, 29, 361–7.

Edwards, B. and Clarke, V. 2004. The psychological impact of a cancer diagnosis on families: the influence of family functioning and patients' illness characteristics on depression and anxiety. *Psycho-Oncology*, 13, 562–76.

Esbensen, B. A., Swane, C. E., Hallberg, I. R. and Thome, B. 2008. Being given a cancer diagnosis in old age: a phenomenological study. *International Journal of Nursing Studies*, 45, 393–405.

Esper, P. and Heidrich, D. 2005. Symptom clusters in advanced illness. *Seminars in Oncology Nursing*, 21, 20–8.

Fan, G., Filipczak, L. and Chow, E. 2007. Symptom clusters in cancer patients: a review of the literature. *Current Oncology*, 14, 173–9.

Fawcett, J. 2005. *Contemporary nursing knowledge: analysis and evaluation of nursing models and theories*, Philadelphia: F.A. Davis.

Ferrell, B., McCabe, M. S. and Levit, L. 2013. The Institute of Medicine report on high-quality cancer care: implications for oncology nursing. *Oncology Nursing Forum*, 40, 603–9.

Frank, A. W. 2003. Survivorship as craft and conviction: reflections on research in progress. *Qualitative Health Research*, 13, 247–55.

Frenkel, M., Ben-Arye, E. and Cohen, L. 2010. Communication in cancer care: discussing complementary and alternative medicine. *Integrative Cancer Therapies*, 9, 177–85.

Geiger, A. M., West, C. N., Nekhlyudov, L., Herrinton, L. J., Liu, I. L., Altschuler, A., Rolnick, S. J., Harris, E. L., Greene, S. M., Elmore, J. G., Emmons, K. M. and Fletcher, S. W.

2006. Contentment with quality of life among breast cancer survivors with and without contralateral prophylactic mastectomy. *Journal of Clinical Oncology*, 24, 1350–6.

Gil, K. M., Mishel, M. H., Belyea, M., Germino, B., Porter, L. S. and Clayton, M. F. 2006. Benefits of the uncertainty management intervention for African American and White older breast cancer survivors: 20-month outcomes. *International Journal of Behavioral Medicine*, 13, 286–94.

Gilbar, O. and Zusman, A. 2007. The correlation between coping strategies, doctor-patient/ spouse relationships and psychological distress among women cancer patients and their spouses. *Psycho-Oncology*, 16, 1010–8.

Grimsbo, G. H., Finset, A. and Ruland, C. M. 2011. Left hanging in the air: experiences of living with cancer as expressed through E-mail communications with oncology nurses. *Cancer Nursing*, 34, 107–16.

Grumann, M. M. and Spiegel, D. 2003. Living in the face of death: interviews with 12 terminally ill women on home hospice care. *Palliative & Supportive Care*, 1, 23–32.

Haase, J. E. 1987. Components of courage in chronically ill adolescents: a phenomenological study. *Advances in Nursing Science*, 9, 64–80.

Hagerty, R. G., Butow, P. N., Ellis, P. M., Lobb, E. A., Pendlebury, S. C., Leighl, N., Macleod, C. and Tattersall, M. H. 2005. Communicating with realism and hope: incurable cancer patients' views on the disclosure of prognosis. *Journal of Clinical Oncology*, 23, 1278–88.

Hamric, A. B., Spross, J. A. and Hanson, C. M. 2014. *Advanced Practice Nursing: An Integrative Approach*. St. Louis: Saunders Elsevier.

Harden, J. K. 2005. Developmental life stage and couples' experiences with prostate cancer: a review of the literature. *Cancer Nursing*, 28, 85–98.

Harrington, S., McGurk, M. and Llewellyn, C. D. 2008. Positive consequences of head and neck cancer: key correlates of finding benefit. *Journal of Psychosocial Oncology*, 26, 43–62.

Henoch, I., Bergman, B. and Danielson, E. 2008. Dyspnea experience and management strategies in patients with lung cancer. *Psycho-Oncology*, 17, 709–15.

Heppner, P. P., Armer, J. M. and Mallinckrodt, B. 2009. Problem-solving style and adaptation in breast cancer survivors: a prospective analysis. *Journal of Cancer Survivorship*, 3, 128–36.

Homs, M. Y., Kuipers, E. J. and Siersema, P. D. 2005. Palliative therapy. *Journal of Surgical Oncology*, 92, 246–56.

Houttekier, D., Cohen, J., Bilsen, J., Addington-Hall, J., Onwuteaka-Philipsen, B. and Deliens, L. 2010. Place of death in metropolitan regions: metropolitan versus non-metropolitan variation in place of death in Belgium, The Netherlands and England. *Health & Place*, 16, 132–9.

Hubbard, G., Kidd, L. and Kearney, N. 2010. Disrupted lives and threats to identity: the experiences of people with colorectal cancer within the first year following diagnosis. *Health (London)*, 14, 131–46.

Institute of Medicine. 2013. *Delivering High-Quality Cancer Care*, ed. by Institute of Medicine. Washington: IOM.

Julkunen, J., Gustavsson-Lilius, M. and Hietanen, P. 2009. Anger expression, partner support, and quality of life in cancer patients. *Journal of Psychosomatic Research*, 66, 235–44.

Kenne Sarenmalm, E., Thoren-Jonsson, A. L., Gaston-Johansson, F. and Ohlen, J. 2009. Making sense of living under the shadow of death: adjusting to a recurrent breast cancer illness. *Qualitative Health Research*, 19, 1116–30.

Khalili, Y. 2007. Ongoing transitions: the impact of a malignant brain tumour on patient and family. *Axone*, 28, 5–13.

Krebsliga Schweiz. 2012. Krebs in der Schweiz: wichtige Zahlen. In Krebsliga Schweiz (ed.), *Krebs in der Schweiz.* Bern: Schweizerische Krebsliga.

Lauver, D. R., Connolly-Nelson, K. and Vang, P. 2007. Stressors and coping strategies among female cancer survivors after treatments. *Cancer Nursing,* 30, 101–11.

Lebel, S., Rosberger, Z., Edgar, L. and Devins, G. M. 2007. Comparison of four common stressors across the breast cancer trajectory. *Journal of Psychosomatic Research,* 63, 225–32.

Ledesma, D. and Kumano, H. 2009. Mindfulness-based stress reduction and cancer: a meta-analysis. *Psycho-Oncology,* 18, 571–9.

Lemay, K. and Wilson, K. G. 2008. Treatment of existential distress in life threatening illness: a review of manualized interventions. *Clinical Psychology Review,* 28, 472–93.

Lovgren, M., Hamberg, K. and Tishelman, C. 2010. Clock time and embodied time experienced by patients with inoperable lung cancer. *Cancer Nursing,* 33, 55–63.

Lynn, J. and Adamson, D. M. 2003. Living well at the End of Life. Adapting health care to serious chronic illness in old age. In RAND (ed.), *RAND Health.* Pittsburgh: RAND.

Manne, S., Badr, H., Zaider, T., Nelson, C. and Kissane, D. 2010. Cancer-related communication, relationship intimacy, and psychological distress among couples coping with localized prostate cancer. *Journal of Cancer Survivorship,* 4, 74–85.

Marcus, A. C., Garrett, K. M., Cella, D. F., Wenzel, L., Brady, M. J., Fairclough, D., Pate-Willig, M., Barnes, D., Emsbo, S. P., Kluhsman, B. C., Crane, L., Sedlacek, S. and Flynn, P. J. 2010. Can telephone counseling post-treatment improve psychosocial outcomes among early stage breast cancer survivors? *Psycho-Oncology,* 19, 923–32.

Martin, J. S., Ummenhofer, W., Manser, T. and Spirig, R. 2010. Interprofessional collaboration among nurses and physicians: making a difference in patient outcome. *Swiss Medical Weekly,* 140, w13062.

McCorkle, R., Dowd, M., Ercolano, E., Schulman-Green, D., Williams, A. L., Siefert, M. L., Steiner, J. and Schwartz, P. 2008. Effects of a nursing intervention on quality of life outcomes in post-surgical women with gynecological cancers. *Psycho-Oncology.*

McCorkle, R., Dowd, M., Ercolano, E., Schulman-Green, D., Williams, A. L., Siefert, M. L., Steiner, J. and Schwartz, P. 2009. Effects of a nursing intervention on quality of life outcomes in post-surgical women with gynecological cancers. *Psycho-Oncology,* 18, 62–70.

McCorry, N. K., Dempster, M., Clarke, C. and Doyle, R. 2009. Adjusting to life after esophagectomy: the experience of survivors and carers. *Qualitative Health Research,* 19, 1485–94.

McMillan, S. C., Small, B. J., Weitzner, M., Schonwetter, R., Tittle, M., Moody, L. and Haley, W. E. 2006. Impact of coping skills intervention with family caregivers of hospice patients with cancer: a randomized clinical trial. *Cancer,* 106, 214–22.

Mehnert, A. 2006. Meaning and spirituality in patients with chronic somatic illness. *Bundesgesundheitsblatt Gesundheitsforschung Gesundheitsschutz,* 49, 780–7.

Mehnert, A., Lehmann, C., Cao, P. and Koch, U. 2006. Assessment of psychosocial distress and resources in oncology – a literature review about screening measures and current developments. *Psychotherapie, Psychosomatik, medizinische Psychologie,* 56, 462–79.

Mellon, S., Kershaw, T. S., Northouse, L. L. and Freeman-Gibb, L. 2007. A family-based model to predict fear of recurrence for cancer survivors and their caregivers. *Psycho-Oncology,* 16, 214–23.

Miaskowski, C. 2006. Symptom clusters: establishing the link between clinical practice and symptom management research. *Supportive Care in Cancer,* 14, 792–4.

Mikulincer, M., Florian, V. and Hirschberger, G. 2003. The existential function of close relationships: introducing death into the science of love. *Personality & Social Psychology Review,* 7, 20–40.

Mishel, M. H. 1981. The measurement of uncertainty in illness. *Nursing Research*, 30, 258–63.

Mishel, M. H. and Clayton, M. F. 2008. Theories of uncertainties in illness. In M. J. Smith and P. R. Liehr (eds.), *Middle Range Theory for Nursing*. New York, NY: Springer.

Mishel, M. H., Germino, B. B., Gil, K. M., Belyea, M., Laney, I. C., Stewart, J., Porter, L. and Clayton, M. F. 2005. Benefits from an uncertainty management intervention for African-American and Caucasian older long-term breast cancer survivors. *Psycho-Oncology*, 14, 962–78.

Moene, M., Bergbom, I. and Skott, C. 2006. Patients' existential situation prior to colorectal surgery. *Journal of Advanced Nursing*, 54, 199–207.

Molassiotis, A., Wengstrom, Y. and Kearney, N. 2010. Symptom cluster patterns during the first year after diagnosis with cancer. *Journal of Pain and Symptom Management*, 39, 847–58.

Mosher, C. E. and Danoff-Berg, S. 2007. Death anxiety and cancer-related stigma: a terror management analysis. *Death Studies*, 31, 885–907.

National Cancer Institute. 2015. *SEER Stat Fact Sheets: All Cancer Sites*. National Cancer Institute.

Nelson, C. J., Weinberger, M. I., Balk, E., Holland, J., Breitbart, W. and Roth, A. J. 2009. The chronology of distress, anxiety, and depression in older prostate cancer patients. *Oncologist*, 14, 891–9.

Northouse, L. L. 2005. Helping families of patients with cancer. *Oncolology Nursing Forum*, 32, 743–50.

Northouse, L. L., Katapodi, M. C., Song, L., Zhang, L. and Mood, D. W. 2010. Interventions with family caregivers of cancer patients: meta-analysis of randomized trials. *Cancer Journal for Clinicians*, 60, 317–39.

Northouse, L. L., Mood, D. W., Schafenacker, A., Montie, J. E., Sandler, H. M., Forman, J. D., Hussain, M., Pienta, K. J., Smith, D. C. and Kershaw, T. 2007. Randomized clinical trial of a family intervention for prostate cancer patients and their spouses. *Cancer*, 110, 2809–18.

OECD Ilibrary. 2015. *Deaths From Cancer* [Online]. Paris-Cedex: OECD iLibrary. [Accessed February 16, 2015].

Paterson, B. L. 2000. "Are we in Kansas yet, Toto?" The construction of chronic illness in research. *Canadian Journal of Nursing Research*, 32, 11–7.

Paterson, B. L. 2001. The shifting perspectives model of chronic illness. *Journal of Nursing Scholarship*, 33, 21–6.

Paterson, B. L. 2003. The koala has claws: applications of the shifting perspectives model in research of chronic illness. *Qualitative Health Research*, 13, 987–94.

Paton, A., Stein, D. E., D'Agostino, R., Pastores, S. M. and Halpern, N. A. 2013. Critical care medicine advanced practice provider model at a comprehensive cancer center: successes and challenges. *American Journal of Critical Care*, 22, 439–43.

Penson, R. T., Partridge, R. A., Shah, M. A., Giansiracusa, D., Chabner, B. A. and Lynch, T. J., Jr. 2005. Fear of death. *Oncologist*, 10, 160–9.

Porter, L. S., Keefe, F. J., Baucom, D. H., Hurwitz, H., Moser, B., Patterson, E. and Kim, H. J. 2009. Partner-assisted emotional disclosure for patients with gastrointestinal cancer: results from a randomized controlled trial. *Cancer*, 115, 4326–38.

Ramfelt, E., Severinsson, E. and Lützén, K. 2002. Attempting to find meaning in illness to achieve emotional coherence: the experiences of patients with colorectal cancer. *Cancer Nursing*, 25, 141–9.

Robinson, P. J. and Wood, K. 1983. Fear of death and physical illness: a personal construct approach. *Death Education*, 7, 213–28.

Rogers, L. Q., Markwell, S., Hopkins-Price, P., Vicari, S., Courneya, K. S., Hoelzer, K. and Verhulst, S. 2011. Reduced barriers mediated physical activity maintenance among breast cancer survivors. *Journal of Sport and Exercise Psychology*, 33, 235–54.

Sanatani, M., Schreier, G. and Stitt, L. 2008. Level and direction of hope in cancer patients: an exploratory longitudinal study. *Supportive Care in Cancer*, 16, 493–9.

Sant, M., Allemani, C., Santaquilani, M., Knijn, A., Marchesi, F. and Capocaccia, R. 2009. EUROCARE-4. Survival of cancer patients diagnosed in 1995–1999. Results and commentary. *European Journal of Cancer*, 45, 931–91.

Sarna, L., Brown, J. K., Cooley, M. E., Williams, R. D., Chernecky, C., Padilla, G. and Danao, L. L. 2005. Quality of life and meaning of illness of women with lung cancer. *Oncology Nursing Forum*, 32, E9–19.

Schulte, A. 2002. Consensus versus disagreement in disease-related stigma: a comparison of reactions to AIDS and cancer patients. *Sociological Perspectives*, 45, 81–104.

Shaha, M. 2003a. *The Omnipresence of Cancer*. Doctoral thesis, City University London.

Shaha, M. 2003b. Life with intestinal cancer. A phenomenologic-empirical study. *Pflege*, 16, 323–30.

Shaha, M. and Bauer-Wu, S. 2009. Early adulthood uprooted: transitoriness in young women with breast cancer. *Cancer Nursing*, 32, 246–55.

Shaha, M. and Cox, C. L. 2003. The omnipresence of cancer. *European Journal of Oncology Nursing*, 7, 191–6.

Shaha, M., Cox, C. L., Belcher, A. E. and Cohen, M. Z. 2011a. Transitoriness: patients' perception of life after a diagnosis of cancer. *Cancer Nursing Practice*, 10, 24–7.

Shaha, M., Cox, C. L., Cohen, M. Z., Belcher, A. E. and Kappeli, S. 2011b. The contribution of concept development to nursing knowledge? The example of Transitoriness. *Pflege*, 24, 361–72.

Shaha, M., Cox, C. L., Hall, A., Porrett, T. and Brown, J. 2006. The omnipresence of cancer: its implications for colorectal cancer. *Cancer Nursing Practice*, 5, 35–9.

Shaha, M., Cox, C. L., Talman, K. and Kelly, D. 2008. Uncertainty in breast, prostate, and colorectal cancer: implications for supportive care. *Journal of Nursing Scholarship*, 40, 60–7.

Shaha, M., Pandian, V., Choti, M. A., Stotsky, E., Herman, J. M., Khan, Y., Libonati, C., Pawlik, T. M., Schulick, R. D. and Belcher, A. E. 2010. Transitoriness in cancer patients: a cross-sectional survey of lung and gastrointestinal cancer patients. *Supportive Care in Cancer*, 19, 271–9.

Sherman, A. C., Simonton, S., Latif, U. and Bracy, L. 2010. Effects of global meaning and illness-specific meaning on health outcomes among breast cancer patients. *Journal of Behavioral Medicine*, 33, 364–77.

Siegel, R., Ma, J., Zou, Z. and Jemal, A. 2014. Cancer statistics, 2014. *CA: A Cancer Journal for Clinicians*, 64, 9–29.

Sigal, J. J., Claude Ouimet, M., Margolese, R., Panarello, L., Stibernik, V. and Bescec, S. 2008. How patients with less-advanced and more-advanced cancer deal with three death-related fears: an exploratory study. *Journal of Psychosocial Oncology*, 26, 53–68.

Simpson, M. F. and Whyte, F. 2006. Patients' experiences of completing treatment for colorectal cancer in a Scottish District General Hospital. *European Journal of Cancer Care*, 15, 172–82.

Stang, I. and Mittelmark, M. B. 2010. Intervention to enhance empowerment in breast cancer self-help groups. *Nursing Inquiry*, 17, 47–57.

Staudacher, D. 2011. Im Schatten der Ungewissheit. Aspekte eines existentiellen Pflegekonzepts. *NOVA Cura*, 42, 14–16.

Steel, J. L., Gamblin, T. C. and Carr, B. I. 2008. Measuring post-traumatic growth in people diagnosed with hepatobiliary cancer: directions for future research. *Oncology Nursing Forum*, 35, 643–50.

Svensson, H., Brandberg, Y., Einbeigi, Z., Hatschek, T. and Ahlberg, K. 2008. Psycho-logical reactions to progression of metastatic breast cancer-an interview study. *Cancer Nursing*, 32, 55–63.

Taubman-Ben-Ari, O., Findler, L. and Mikulincer, M. 2002. The effects of mortality salience on relationship strivings and beliefs: the moderating role of attachment style. *British Journal of Social Psychology*, 41, 419–41.

Thompson, G. N., Chochinov, H. M., Wilson, K. G., McPherson, C. J., Chary, S., O'Shea, F. M., Kuhl, D. R., Fainsinger, R. L., Gagnon, P. R. and MacMillan, K. A. 2009. Prog-nostic acceptance and the well-being of patients receiving palliative care for cancer. *Journal of Clinical Oncology*, 27, 5757–62.

Timmermans, L. M., Van Zuuren, F. J., Van der Maazen, R. W., Leer, J. W. and Kraaimaat, F. W. 2007. Monitoring and blunting in palliative and curative radiotherapy consulta-tions. *Psycho-Oncology*, 16, 1111–20.

Vollmer, T. C., Wittmann, M., Schweiger, C. and Hiddemann, W. 2011. Preoccupation with death as predictor of psychological distress in patients with haematologic malignancies. *European Journal of Cancer Care*, 20, 403–11.

Wallston, K. A. 2005. The validity of the multidimensional health locus of control scales. *Journal of Health Psychology*, 10, 623–31.

Weaver, L. C., Jessup, A. and Mayer, D. K. 2013. Cancer survivorship care: implications for primary care advanced practice nurses. *Nurse Practitioners*, 38, 1–11.

Westman, B., Bergenmar, M. and Andersson, L. 2006. Life, illness and death – existential reflections of a Swedish sample of patients who have undergone curative treatment for breast or prostatic cancer. *European Journal of Oncology Nursing*, 10, 169–76.

WHO. 2014. *Fact Sheet N° 297. Cancer* [Online]. Geneva: World Health Organization. Available at: www.who.int/mediacentre/factsheets/fs297/en/index.html#. [Accessed March 28, 2014].

Wonghongkul, T., Dechaprom, N., Phumivichuvate, L. and Losawatkul, S. 2006. Uncer-tainty appraisal coping and quality of life in breast cancer survivors. *Cancer Nursing*, 29, 250–7.

5   Ethical dimensions of the theory

The Omnipresence of Cancer

M. Zumstein-Shaha and V. Tschudin

Introduction

Healthcare is expected to be good practice, integrating the latest evidence. Good practice is also based on and guided by theory[1] (McEwen and Wills, 2007). Thus, interprofessional practice, the development and growth of clinical experience and self-reflection are promoted (Benner, 2001; Grace and Milliken, 2016). Subsequently healthcare involves the best course of action taken by professionals who have a basis for decision making or providing adequate care (Grace and Milliken, 2016; McEwen and Wills, 2007; McKenna et al., 2015). Given the increase of elderly people in our society and as a result, an augmentation of the group of patients suffering from chronic diseases and acute diseases such as cancer, often presenting with complex illness situations; theory-guided practice is no longer an option, but a must. As part of theory-guided practice, ethical considerations are key. Healthcare professionals not only need a sound ethical basis consisting of knowledge of ethical theories and principles, they also need theories that are expected to guide practice. These theories need to consist of a sound basis that include ethical considerations. In order to select suitable theories that fulfil these requirements, analysis of existing theories is needed.

The theory analysis proposed by McEwen and Wills (2007) involves identification of existing standards of care, congruence with existing nursing interventions and therapeutics and the societal and cross-cultural relevance of a theory. Thus, theories guiding practice are expected to fulfil certain criteria.

For the selection of a theory and determining its use for practice, values, beliefs and attitudes point to the ethical dimension of a theory. Therefore, exploring these values, beliefs and attitudes will help healthcare professionals identify the ethical basis and the practice that may emerge from a chosen theory. Not only is the exploration of a theory's underlying basis necessary to know the ethical dimension; this will also help healthcare professionals determine their own and the theory's stated identity. McKenna et al. (2015: 144) maintain that '[t]he selection of a nursing theory is value-laden'. Choosing a theory is therefore already influenced by the values, beliefs and attitudes of those who execute the selection. Subsequently, the ethical (societal, social) and moral (personal) elements of any selected theory need to be identified to determine its use in practice. Many tools exist to analyse and evaluate a theory (McKenna et al., 2015; McEwen and Wills, 2007; Fawcett and Desanto-Madeya, 2013; Smith and Parker, 2015). Theory analysis allows for the identification of the purpose and the scope of the theory, its key concepts, underlying values and its link to practice. Smith and Parker (2015: 23ff) propose several questions to identify the values of the respective nursing staff, practice and theory. Theory-guided practice is only possible and meaningful if the underlying values of any given theory can be adopted by the healthcare professionals who will use it (Smith and Parker, 2015). In order to identify these values, the following questions are suggested:

- What nursing theory seems consistent with the values and beliefs that guide my practice?
- What theories are consistent with my personal values and beliefs?
- What do I hope to achieve from the use of nursing theory?
- Given my reflection on a nursing situation, how can I use theory to support this description of my practice?
- How can I use nursing theory to improve my practice for myself and for the patients in my care?

(Smith and Parker, 2015: 30)[2]

In their set of criteria for theory evaluation, Smith and Parker (2015) ask about the actions that constitute nursing within any given theory. Other questions include the distinctions between other healthcare professions included in the possible use of a theory, as well as the underlying vision of nursing in this theory. Smith and Parker (2015) ask about the relevance of the theory for the institutions in which nursing takes place. These questions can be useful in determining a suitable theory for guiding healthcare. While the theory has to be based on ethical understanding and social norms, the process of analysing the theory also has to be ethical. In concentrating on the process as an exercise in professional ethical behaviour, a vital work of learning is taking place by initially clarifying personal and professional values, beliefs and attitudes in order to use ethical processes competently.

Care takes place between patients and healthcare professionals as part of a relationship that is being created at this moment, and which should in theory be, 'patient-centred and collaborative' (Armstrong, 2006: 112). The patient-healthcare professional relationship constitutes an essential element of theories in nursing. Within such relationships, healthcare professionals, and in particular nurses, have three main roles. One role includes recovery after treatments, support of survivorship and health promotion. Another role promotes self-care to facilitate returning to everyday life. A third role relates to the end of life, which includes advanced symptom management, palliation and working towards maintaining dignity and a dignified death (Armstrong, 2006). The patients' personal values, beliefs and attitudes and the ethical approaches used in care by nurses and other healthcare professionals are therefore important elements of this relationship (Armstrong, 2006; Tschudin, 2003a; Tschudin, 2003b). The ethical aspects of the theory *The Omnipresence of Cancer* are explored in this chapter in order to determine its relevance for the healthcare professional-patient relationship.

Background

Ethical knowing

Tschudin (2003a: preface ix) states that [a]ll nursing practice is ethical practice'. Similarly, Held (2006: 42) states that, care is both a practice and a value'. Caring practice encompasses the identification and development of suitable actions as responses to patients' needs. Care as a basic value refers to and emphasises the patient-healthcare professional relationship (Held, 2006) and therefore the interactions between patients and healthcare professionals need to be, and to be seen to be, ethical care (Tschudin, 2003a: preface viii). Ethical knowing is thus introduced as an important element of a theory that may be applicable to practice. Ethical knowing is growing in importance for nursing and healthcare professionals because of increasing demands on healthcare by growing numbers of elderly people with multiple needs, increasing financial constraints on the population, a growing lack of well-educated and trained healthcare professionals and, as a result, less and less time to care for patients and their families (Smith and Parker, 2015; Institute of Medicine, 2010; Institute of Medicine, 2013).

For a theory to be useful in practice, it does not only need to describe phenomena that guide practice, but it also needs to address healthcare and/or nursing care, in particular, the healthcare professional-patient relationship, and be transparent about underlying values, attitudes and beliefs.

To describe essential knowledge for practice, five different 'patterns of knowing' have been described in nursing (Chinn and Kramer, 2015; Carper, 1978; White, 1995). Each one of these patterns circumscribes an area of specific knowledge, which contributes important information for nurses to care for their patients. In practice, the knowledge intersects and overlaps in order for nursing to be best patient-centred practice (Chinn and Kramer, 2015).

For nursing theory to be meaningful for practice, it is important that the use of the theory will enhance the five patterns of knowing that produce specific knowledge useful for care. To date, however, the type of knowledge produced by nursing theories has rarely been explored. In particular, ethical knowing being produced by a theory has only marginally been addressed (Shaha, 2014). One way of considering ethical knowing has been proposed by Bergum (1994). According to Bergum (1994), ethical knowing includes descriptive, abstract and inherent knowledge.

As with the patterns of knowing described by Chinn and Kramer (Table 5.1), the knowledge types proposed by Bergum (1994) also intersect, overlap and do not exist in isolation. All three knowledge types are essential in order to be representative of the whole person of the patient and the healthcare professional

Table 5.1 Ways of knowing

Pattern	Description
Empirical knowing	Knowledge related to evidence-based practice.
	Development of theories to guide research, education and practice.
Personal knowing	Knowledge related to the individual, be it patients or healthcare professionals.
	Identification and clarification of values, beliefs and attitudes.
Aesthetic knowing	Experiential knowing in combination with reflective thinking, which allows for professional growth.
	Instinctively know the best action to improve patients' situation.
Ethical knowing	Knowledge of ethical theories, principles and codes of conduct.
	Development and fostering of human values and dignity to provide ethical care to patients and their families.
Emancipatory knowing	Knowledge related to the societal and political environment of health care.
	Influence of healthcare professionals by their surroundings, i.e., space, room and climate.

Legend: This table is adapted from Carper, 1978 and Chinn and Kramer (2015).

Table 5.2 Knowledge description and patterns of knowing

Knowledge	Description	Patterns of knowing
Descriptive	A narrative account from patients about the illness situation, the associated emotions, reflections and considerations is obtained.	Personal, aesthetic and emancipatory knowledge
Abstract	Abstract knowledge is developed through research, following systematic procedures, scientifically accepted methods and ethical standards. As part of holistic care, abstract knowledge is the link between descriptive knowledge and existing evidence.	Empirical knowledge
Inherent	Inherent knowledge refers to relationships between persons. As part of the patient-healthcare professional relationship, healthcare professionals try to get to know the patients and relate this knowledge to descriptive and abstract knowledge.	Ethical (and aesthetic) knowledge

Legend: Adapted from Bergum (1994) and Chinn and Kramer (2015).

Table 5.3 Knowledge production and description

Knowledge production	Description
Dominance to collaboration	Developing ethical knowledge as identified by Bergum (1994: 76), needs to be preceded by the specific and inherent knowledge provided by the patient. Professionals are asked to collaborate with patients and their experiences.
Abstraction to context	In order to make sense of a given situation, it is necessary to include knowledge about the context, as well as the personal account of the patient. This includes not only the physical context, but also the political and societal environment in which an illness situation occurs.
Beneficence to nurturance	With this part, the idea of collaboration is reinforced. Professionals are asked to engage authentically in the relationship with the patient. There is a demand to 'share the patient's journey' (Bergum, 1994: 78).

Legend: This table is adapted from Bergum (1994).

(Bergum, 1994). Knowledge for ethical care is produced in three ways: from 'dominance to collaboration', from 'abstraction to context' and from 'beneficence to nurturance'.

Ethical knowing therefore needs to include the means of enabling the personal narrative to be told by (or about) patients, and the personal and professional knowledge of the practitioner, including intuitive, contextual and societal knowledge. Ethical knowing starts with a thorough understanding of personal standards and values held, professional codes of conduct, ethical theories and the various approaches to a situation that need to be considered in order to achieve resolution.

Philosophical bases

The traditional broad theories of ethics in western philosophy are utilitarianism and deontology. Utilitarianism emerged from the works of the philosophers Jeremy Bentham (1748–1832) and John Stuart Mill (1806–1873), who stated that a human action is evaluated as right or wrong in consideration of its potential consequences or the respective objective (DeGrazia and Brand-Ballard, 2011). The theory concentrates on the outcome of an action, that is, a person's actions are morally right if their consequences contribute to the well-being of others. Hence, a person's actions are expected to produce as much happiness as another action by another person at the same time. In relation to a theory such as *The Omnipresence of Cancer*, the means of care and treatment and how they are carried out are of less importance than the final outcome, which would be expected to be fully satisfying. In short, the end justifies the means.

The theory more commonly applied in healthcare is deontology, or duty theory. All codes of ethics are based on this theory. The most well-known theory that focuses on duties is that outlined by Immanuel Kant (1724–1894). Deontological theories explore what is morally right or wrong in an action itself; not necessarily its consequences. According to Kant, there is only one concept of a morally right action, known as the 'categorical imperative': 'Act only according to that maxim whereby you can at the same time will that it should become a universal law without contradiction' (DeGrazia and Brand-Ballard, 2011: 18; Kant, 1986: Grounding of the metaphysics of morals: 117; universalizability principle). All healthcare professionals owe a duty of care to patients, and in any difficulties or disputes, the main concern is always how this was carried out or interpreted at the time. In short, the means matter, not the end result.

There are many other basic philosophies of ethics, especially those well-known from other cultures. Asian and Eastern philosophies are based on compassion (from a Buddhist basis) and the life-long attempt to eliminate suffering. Philosophies and theories based on Islamic foundations concentrate on the duty to obey the laws, or to 'submit' to the laws by doing certain acts, always anticipating the final judgement. The African concept of 'Ubuntu' is variously translated as human kindness, humanity towards others or, practically, as 'I am a human being because you are a human being'. Many Indigenous societies, e.g., in the Americas, Australia and New Zealand, have lived by their philosophical and religious bases for centuries, and each of their systems is valid and 'right' in their own context and practice. It is not expected that healthcare professionals are conversant with the details of such ways of life, but that they acknowledge and respect them.

None of the basic theories and philosophies can be applied exclusively to a situation, as has sometimes been maintained. In practice, every situation is unique, with many differing aspects rising and falling away in the course of an illness trajectory. In practice, all ethical theories overlap, are partly applicable and relevant. Hence the need to be knowledgeable about their relevance and usefulness in any given situation.

Different ways of approaching ethics can be considered as theories in themselves, often also known as moral theories. Some approaches (e.g., feminist ethics) are disputed as being theories in themselves, but each in their own way attempts to provide a 'reasoned response to practical questions such as "How should we live?" or "What should we do?" asked of matters ranging from the public and political to the intimate and domestic' (O'Neill, 1991). Some of the best-known such theories are care ethics, virtue ethics, feminist ethics, narrative ethics and principle-based ethics.

Care ethics

Care is more basic than medicine. Care goes on long after interventions or treatments have been given. Thus, care is life-enhancing in a more profound way than medicine is. Nightingale based all her work on care and how it is given, and she took it for granted that the women who became nurses knew instinctively how to care.

Table 5.4 Components of caring and definitions

Components of caring	Definition
Compassion	A way of living born out of an awareness of one's relationship to all living creatures.
Competence	A state of having knowledge, judgement, skills, energy, experience and motivation required to respond adequately to the demands of one's professional responsibilities.
Confidence	The quality that fosters trusting relationships.
Conscience	A state of moral awareness, a compass directing one's behaviour according to the moral fitness of things.
Commitment	A complex affective response characterised by a convergence between one's desires and one's obligations and by a deliberate choice to act in accordance with them.
Comportment	Dress and language are symbols of communication in a caring presence.

Legend: This table is adapted from Roach's '5C's/6C's' of caring (Roach, 2002).

Table 5.5 Components of care

Caring about	Worrying about someone or something. This corresponds to the ethical attitude of attention.
Taking care of	Looking after or providing care. One takes responsibility for improving the condition of the other.
Caregiving	Carrying out the care.
Care receiving	The focus is on the patient or care-receiver, who has to be able to respond to the care with feedback, even with 'thank you'.

Legend: This table reflects Tronto's Comportments of Care (Gastmans, 2006: 136–137).

Researcher Sister Simone Roach first moved the subject 'care' from theory to 'a way of being'. She believed that caring is common to all humanity but uniquely expressed through nursing (Roach, 1984). She had the foresight to detail what this meant in practice and developed the 'Five C's of caring', later adding a sixth 'C', comportment (Roach, 2002).

Tronto (1993) first set out a detailed account of the characteristics of care, almost as a summary of the research by Kohlberg (1981) and Gilligan (1982), Noddings (1984) and others. Tronto (1993) distinguished four components of care, rather than giving a specific definition of it.

A brief description of aspects of values will complement these considerations.

VALUES

Most nurses will be familiar with Maslow's Hierarchy of Needs (1970), detailing the values deemed necessary for psychological well-being. Values are seen as 'the personal aspects and foundations of social and ethical living' (Tschudin,

2003b: 27), with virtues (see below) being the visible expressions of the values held. Holding a value of compassion will express itself in showing compassion in relevant situations. Levels of expression of values fall into beliefs, attitudes and values themselves.

Personal and social values change throughout life. They are formed after specific experiences of life (e.g., the birth of a (disabled) child) or in nature (a beautiful sunset). Social values change constantly (e.g., accepting homosexuality as a norm, concern for and contributing to environmental issues), and society is changed by them. Values are more given than chosen.

Essential in care ethics is that everyone concerned with a care situation is considered as equal and has an equal role in giving and taking. Patients receive and give, and carers receive and give. This theory is therefore particularly appropriate to consider in situations, e.g., where relationships cause problems, or families, children, intimacy or particularly personal issues are at stake.

BELIEFS

Beliefs are the most basic level and start from some fact. Anne Frank, the German-born Jewish girl, known from her diary written while hiding from the Nazis during the Second World War and who died in Bergen-Belsen concentration camp, aged 15, wrote, 'I keep my ideals, because in spite of everything I still believe that people are really good at heart' (Frank, 1954). Beliefs are also the oldest level. The belief that the earth is round and not flat took centuries to change.

ATTITUDES

'Some of the attitudes particular to nursing are expressed in the way care is given' (Tschudin, 2003b: 28). A well-known criticism of today's care is often that it is given unwillingly, in a hurry or without due attention to the care-recipient. Attitudes of caring by paying attention to the person can matter as much as the care given itself and arise out of the values held.

Virtue ethics

In most situations of urgency or dilemma, the first question is normally 'what should I do?' Virtue ethics considers this as secondary to the question 'who is the good man or woman?' Asking this first 'then deepens into consideration of those moral qualities (virtues) that might be required' (de Raeve, 2006: 97–98) in a given situation. Rather than concentrating on rights and wrongs or assessing consequences of actions, virtue ethics starts by considering what is there in the way of qualities of the people concerned. Nightingale simply said that 'a good nurse must be a good woman' (Nightingale, 1879). She goes on, 'And how is a good woman to be made and kept?' (Nightingale, 1879). With this question she immediately touches on the crux of virtue ethics: seeking the moral exemplar for education and maintenance of virtue in healthcare professionals. Nightingale's own answer was '. . . a nurse is (A) to be sober and chaste, (B) strictly honest and true, and (C) kind and devoted' (Nightingale, 1879: 475). Today's choice of words would perhaps be (A) willing to learn and change one's mind, (B) demonstrate integrity and (C) kind and committed.

Virtue ethics is based on the work of the Greek philosopher Aristotle (384–322 BCE) who detailed the virtues necessary for understanding and pursuing the 'good life', which he considered to be rational people's main aim in life. For this to come about, 'courage' was of most importance. To understand virtue and 'good' is a constant exercise of self-examination and that of the world around one. Big philosophical themes, such as love, beauty, truth, have to be discussed and will always reveal new insights and understanding (see Murdoch, 1970).The virtues are learned in acting virtuously, and in acting virtuously, the desire for understanding them better grows.

The aim of any kind of modern healthcare is simply and explicitly to achieve a good quality of life ('good life') for everyone, and this requires courage of all healthcare professionals in their attitudes, beliefs, values and practice. How these are to be expressed in practice is considered when specific aspects of this theory are questioned in everyday healthcare work.

Feminist ethics

Feminist ethics is not specifically for women or against men, but feminist concerns are about 'the moral wrongs of oppression and domination' (Liaschenko and Peter, 2003: 37); hence, feminist ethics 'addresses these wrongs in all of their manifestations, including those of race, class, disability, sexual orientation and so forth' (Liaschenko and Peter, 2003: 37). Feminist ethics is in constant flux and is also closely allied to care ethics, but because of its awareness of cultural and political situations and movements, issues of trust play a large role. In short, this approach to ethics is mainly concerned with any issue of power, whatever the source. This includes both power used and power not used, or abused. Any situation of ill health is replete with possibilities and sources of dominance and subversion, one simple example being the image of a patient *lying* in bed and a healthcare professional *standing* by the bed. Power itself is neutral, but if power is used to promote human flourishing, then it is used ethically. In this approach to ethics the healthcare professionals' knowledge and conscious practice of attitudes, beliefs, values, and virtues of attention, trust, perception, empathy and awareness of the meanings of relationships and illness are crucial.

Narrative ethics

Narrative – story – has always played a major role in understanding a situation that presents difficulty or even a dilemma. Narrative as ethics therefore considers how stories are told, heard and understood. Most ethics teaching uses examples of events and experiences. Much research is based on qualitative interviews, building an understanding of needs and remedies.

For stories to have the impact necessary, the first requirement is that they can be told and are not suppressed. If a story needs to be told, the climate has to be such that someone is listening with empathy and without prejudice. There needs to be trust in the relationship, i.e., the hearer needs to know what to do with the story and how and when to keep it going, keep it confidential, to whom and how it is disclosed and dealing with ambiguity in the narrative and the relationship.

In his book *The responsible self,* Niebuhr (1963: 67) considered that the urgent question in any situation is, first of all, 'What is happening?' In most circumstances of uncertainty or doubt, the instinctive questions are normally 'what do I need to do?' or 'what do I need to say?' Given the examples of the main characteristics of various ethical approaches, the question 'what is happening?' touches on care and the kind of care given and received, on what or who a good person is and on how the good life is achieved, on how issues of power influence and guide actions and how principles guide thinking; the first step is always hearing a story.

Niebuhr (1963: 67) considered that from earliest times, when people were confronted with issues of controversy or philosophy, they did not ask 'what is the goal?' [or] 'what is the law?', but 'what is happening?' and then 'what is the fitting response to what is happening?' These two questions may need to be asked and answered repeatedly so that a story can develop and the 'truth' gradually emerge.

An ethic of narrative – attention to the how, why, where, when and what of any situation – underlies all true enquiry, and while this seems obvious, it is necessary to make it obvious. Only when a story is 'heard' can it be really dealt with.

Principle-based ethics

In the early 1970s, Beauchamp and Childress were charged with creating a set of principles for biomedical use. These were first published in 1979 (Beauchamp and Childress). These principles were initially hailed as absolute and sufficient, but were soon challenged and even dismissed (DuBose et al., 1994). However, they remain a useful set of guidelines intended for medicine, not nursing, where they tend to be rather too rigid. One particular critique of the four principles of biomedicine is that they are not based on a specific philosophy or cultural framework. Each principle is perceived as a 'prima facie' condition, meaning that each has to be seen as a form of duty to be adhered to.

AUTONOMY

In healthcare, any treatment and care of sick persons needs to uphold and promote their right for autonomy. No treatment or care should be contrary to or limit the patients' exercise of autonomy (Beauchamp and Childress, 2013; DeGrazia and Brand-Ballard, 2011). This perspective is inherent within the nursing theory *The Omnipresence of Cancer.* Similarly, the autonomy of the professionals is to be upheld, but that is a more difficult topic to accept and not strictly dealt with in biomedicine even now.

NON-MALEFICENCE

Any treatment or care carried out in the health system should not produce additional harm for patients (Beauchamp and Childress, 2013; DeGrazia and Brand-Ballard, 2011). A doctor's basic instruction is always 'First, do no harm' and is a dictum dating back to the Hippocratic Oath.

BENEFICENCE

Any kind of actions undertaken during treatment and care should contribute to improve patient health or well-being (Beauchamp and Childress, 2013; DeGrazia and Brand-Ballard, 2011). This perspective as well is evident within the theory *The Omnipresence of Cancer.* This principle, and that of non-maleficence, are often considered as being either equal or even the same, one expressed positively and the other negatively.

JUSTICE

Resources, advantages and disadvantages of treatments and care need to be distributed in an equal and just manner in health care. This aspect is increasingly causing dissatisfaction and problems for all health carers because of social and financial inequalities in society (Beauchamp and Childress, 2013; DeGrazia and Brand-Ballard, 2011) and because of increasingly limited resources of goods and people.

None of the four principles is considered superior to the other. The principles are applied according to the needs of the situation. Hence, the situation determines the principle that is most adequate. To identify the problems and respective or adequate solutions, a situation is analysed with the help of the selected principle (Beauchamp and Childress, 2013; DeGrazia and Brand-Ballard, 2011).

It is noteworthy that these biomedical principles do not include honesty or truth-telling, which is, however, a crucial aspect of medicine. It can be argued that if the principles are upheld, truth is necessarily included. Another item to be aware of is that 'justice' can quickly be understood as 'law' and become a matter of legal process. The law can be seen as 'black-and-white' in practice, whereas ethics always deals with the 'grey' areas and issues at the boundaries of the accepted or unacceptable, the known and the not-yet-known.

Ethical knowing, then, encompasses the importance of having the personal and direct narrative account of the patient, the personal knowledge by the healthcare professional about personal values, attitudes and beliefs as well as means for incorporating aspects of context and society. In addition, ethical knowing needs to include knowledge about existing professional codes, and knowledge about traditional ethical theories and principles. All ethics demands collaboration, inclusion of context and nurturance. Developing ethical knowing needs to be seen as a process where increasing clarity, respect and common understanding of aims strengthen the persons concerned. Grounded in ethical knowing, healthcare professionals aim at 'doing good'. They need to position themselves for support, with the objective of human flourishing.

Discussion

In order to determine the ethical dimension of the theory *The Omnipresence of Cancer*, the approach by Smith and Parker (2015) will be considered, followed by the ethical knowing aspects introduced by Chinn and Kramer (2015) and Bergum (1994).

Partial theory analysis and discussion guided by Smith and Parker (2015)

Smith and Parker (2015) ask about the values and beliefs that are proposed in a theory. For the translation of a theory into practice, these values and beliefs need to be compared with the values and beliefs of the healthcare professionals of the respective practice area and be compatible. In this way, the ethical dimension of a theory can be determined. In the theory *The Omnipresence of Cancer*, values and beliefs are not mentioned directly. However, Heidegger's philosophy is an influential part of the theory. This philosophy maintains that human beings are part of a specific context, and the context is part of people's lives. People are part of networks of other people with whom they interact or even not. Also, people have a history, which in turn influences their potential future. As such, people are adapting to the challenges that are present in life depending on the respective history and the context. Persons are indivisible; a holistic perspective is therefore needed to grasp the whole of human life (Shaha, 2003; Shaha, 2014; Shaha and Cox, 2003).

As the theory focuses on healthcare, values concerning health or illness and the healthcare context need to be present. Persons with a cancer diagnosis, or who have been diagnosed with another life-threatening illness, are at the centre of the theory of *The Omnipresence of Cancer*. The patients continue to live as before, but previous experiences and resources are important to manage their lives with cancer or when facing the end of life. Based on these givens, patients find ways of living with cancer (Shaha, 2014; Gaillard Desmedt and Shaha, 2013).

Healthcare is related to this particular situation, implying a lengthy disease trajectory that eventually ends in a person's death. During this trajectory, many different healthcare actions in the forms of treatments or care are necessary and are provided by many different protagonists. The theory does not differentiate according to the stage of the disease trajectory, but highlights that persons with a life-threatening illness face comprehensive treatments involving complex care that go beyond hospitalisation. The roles of the various healthcare professionals are implicit, but not usually explicitly stated. The main focus is on the persons with life-threatening illnesses who enter health care to have treatment. Detailing the trajectory of life-threatening diseases and the accompanying challenges that people encounter need to be added to the trajectory as they arise. The roles of healthcare professionals across the disease trajectory need also to be described in more detail as the trajectory moves forward.

The care given by nurses and other healthcare professionals is essential for patients and families to navigate through the experience of being diagnosed with a life-threatening disease. Nurses offer the support to patients so that they can integrate the disease into their lives and adjust to this new situation (Shaha, 2014). It is always important to help patients and their families to live their lives despite the life-limiting disease that has come to the fore. The theory provides a way to think about thoughts of death, and also think early within the disease trajectory about the end of life (Shaha, 2014; Shaha et al., 2011).

In summary, the theory provides some values, particularly components of caring mentioned by Roach (2002) or Tronto (1993) (see above). However, detailing them further can be helpful to facilitate translation into practice. Hence, the relevance of the theory is also increased.

Partial theory analysis and discussion guided by ethical knowing as proposed by Chinn and Kramer (2015)

For nursing practice, a theory needs to provide guidance regarding the five patterns of knowing (empirical knowing, personal knowing, aesthetic knowing, ethical knowing, emancipatory knowing) (Chinn and Kramer, 2015) described above.

Table 5.6 Five patterns of knowing

Patterns of knowing	Their representations in theories	The indications within The Omnipresence of Cancer
Empirical knowing	– Propositions for formulating research hypotheses or questions.	– Several propositions are offered, e. g.,: *The Omnipresence of Cancer* constitutes the outcome of the reactions and the experience of being diagnosed with cancer (Shaha, 2014: 126).
Personal knowing	– Underlying values, beliefs and attitudes – Reference to ways of applying self-reflection personally and with others to identify the values, beliefs and attitudes of healthcare professionals, patients and their families.	– Values, beliefs and attitudes are indicated through the prominent role of Heidegger's Ontology of Dasein. – Reference to self-reflection is provided in that the healthcare professionals are expected to be prepared and educated to provide support to patients and their families (Shaha, 2014: 137).
Aesthetic knowing	– Knowledge on intuition.	– Intuition is implicitly considered, e.g., as interventions such as calming and relaxation techniques are recommended (Shaha, 2014: 131).
Ethical knowing	– Knowledge of ethical theories and principles. – Knowledge of professional codes of ethics and/or conducts.	– Ethical theories, principles and codes are addressed explicitly as healthcare professionals are expected to have an ethically sensitive and mature attitude (Shaha, 2014: 138).
Emancipatory knowing.	– Indication of socio-political aspects of care.	– Socio-political aspects are introduced with reference to advanced practice roles in healthcare (Shaha, 2014: 140).

Legend: The five patterns of knowing (Chinn and Kramer, 2015) and their representation in the theory of *The Omnipresence of Cancer*.

Ideally, these five patterns of knowing need to be identifiable within the theory. To facilitate practice implementation, the theory needs to provide guidance on the production of each of these five patterns of knowing.

Healthcare professionals need to be knowledgeable about treatment effects, side effects and sequelae from the treatments or the disease. This is essential in order to guide and provide tailored education for self-management and symptom management by patients and their families. Drawing on existing evidence-based guidelines and standards to assess patients' anxiety, fears of change, uncertainty, dealing with spiritual needs and quality of life is crucial for professionals to respond to patients' needs. The theory is congruent with and supports state-of-the-art interventions. The theory also introduces the concept of Transitoriness, which directly relates to the end of life and end-of-life care (Shaha, 2003; Shaha and Cox, 2003; Shaha et al., 2011; Shaha et al., 2010; Da Rocha et al., 2014). With this concept, thoughts about death and planning for the end of life are introduced, as well as issues about death anxiety, advanced care planning and specific palliative care issues such as 'do not resuscitate (DNR)', nutrition and artificial feeding at the end of life, terminal sedations, euthanasia, and 'letting die'. However, the detailed relationships of all these themes within the theory require further exploration through research. One specific instrument to assess Transitoriness, which these elements signify, is presently being tested (refer to Chapter 6.).

Although an exploration for each of the five patterns of knowing can be carried further, the focus here is on ethical knowing. In nursing, ethical knowing includes knowledge of some guiding ethical theories and the binding professional codes of conduct. The theory is consistent with professional codes, although a detailed statement has yet to be added. Identifying ethical problems constitutes an important part of ethical knowing. At a first and basic level, it is important for professionals to recognize if a situation presents itself primarily as one of care, ethics, law or other dimensions. Being able to clarify these elements enables the involved parties to further the process more easily and clearly. Specific clinical knowledge of the experience of being diagnosed and living with cancer is necessary so that nurses are able to develop and implement adequate support for patients and their families. However, ethical knowledge underlies the evidence and the specific clinical knowledge. This indicates that baccalaureate, masters and doctoral level education is implicitly considered essential for this theory. In this way it will be possible to develop and implement tailored and evidence-based support for patients and families across the disease trajectory and beyond hospital care (Shaha, 2014).

Collaborative work between all healthcare professionals involved in the care of patients (and their families) with cancer or any life-threatening disease is important. Only in this way can knowledge be maximised and comprehensive care be provided to patients and their families throughout the disease trajectory (Shaha et al., 2010).

Partial theory analysis and discussion guided by ethical theories and principles

The philosophical theories of utilitarianism and deontology are not specifically mentioned in the theory, but they are implied. The theory supports healthcare professionals to consider the consequences of their actions in carrying out their duties to patients and their families.

The two dimensions of 'Toward Authentic Dasein' and 'Mapping Out The Future' are parts of the theory. When considering the first dimension, it is relevant to be aware that people are thrown off their equilibrium and more or less consciously transfer their control of the situation to healthcare professionals.

However, this transfer is partial and temporary. As soon as patients are able to grasp the situation again, they regain control. This is linked to the principle of autonomy (Beauchamp and Childress, 2013) and also to feminist ethics, with patients regaining their individual control consciously and deliberately. The theory does require healthcare professionals to consider their own resources of knowledge and experience and distribute them equally among patients and families.

Partial theory analysis and discussion guided by care

The theory's central value is that patients matter and that because their experiences matter to patients, they matter in nursing care (Tschudin, 1999). To provide holistic care for patients and their families, it is essential to draw on the patients' narrative of their disease and life experience, which constitutes ethical knowing. This makes it possible to develop tailored interventions (Shaha, 2003; Shaha and Cox, 2003; Shaha et al., 2011; Shaha et al., 2010; Shaha, 2014).

Descriptive knowledge, as proposed by Bergum (1994: 72–73), is present in the theory in that the narrative of patients' experiences is crucial to understanding the encounter with cancer. It is important that the patients can openly relate their thoughts and feelings. The patients' values, beliefs and attitudes need to be understood to determine the important areas of intervention. These are not necessarily constant, but as the illness or recovery progresses, new narratives come to light and new narratives need to be told and heard. Such experiences are expected to be told to healthcare professionals. In turn, they are expected to be able to clarify *this* particular experience with the repeated questions 'what is happening?' and 'what is the fitting answer?' (Tschudin, 2003b; Shaha, 2003; Shaha and Bauer-Wu, 2009; Shaha and Cox, 2003; Shaha et al., 2008).

The second type of knowledge proposed by Bergum (1994: 73) relates to integrating empirical findings, standards and guidelines with the personal accounts of the patients, making it possible to identify the precise problems associated with the disease. Healthcare professionals are expected to demonstrate a holistic approach to the entire account and thus integrate empirical findings in order to counter-balance fragmentation and possible misunderstanding. In order to demonstrate this holistic approach, skilled professionals can demonstrate the use of one or more ethical theories or approaches in the way that care plans are constructed and followed.

The inherent knowledge identified as necessary by Bergum (1994: 73–74) is gained by having an understanding of what being a patient means, the disease situation and the environment in which this happens. Only through a sincere patient-healthcare professional relationship is it possible to obtain the level of understanding necessary for inherent knowledge. In this relationship, patients and healthcare professionals invest themselves deeply, thus reinforcing the components of care proposed by Roach (2002) and Tronto (1993) (see above). The theory of *The Omnipresence of Cancer* specifically mentions that healthcare professionals engage in a relationship with patients. Further areas of inherent knowledge in the theory need yet to be explored.

The theory states that it is expected that healthcare professionals not only listen to patients and their experiences, but also help them to talk about them (Shaha, 2003; Shaha and Bauer-Wu, 2009; Shaha and Cox, 2003; Shaha et al., 2006; Shaha et al., 2010; Shaha et al., 2011; Shaha, 2014). Care is best provided by interprofessional collaborative healthcare teams. The process 'from beneficence to nurturance' (Bergum, 1994: 77ff) is clearly addressed in this way. It is taken for granted that healthcare professionals aim at providing good care to patients, with the aim of achieving a good quality of life or, in Aristotelian terms, simply the 'good life' (see above). The theory requires healthcare professionals to have current and comprehensive knowledge of health, disease, treatments and potential sequelae or other consequences in relation to potentially life-limiting diseases. Healthcare professionals are also expected to have sufficient knowledge to engage in a therapeutic relationship with patients and their families in order to provide 'adequate and tailored care' (Shaha, 2014: 140).

In summary, the theory addresses many values and beliefs implicitly. However, Heidegger's philosophy is also an important influence, which determines many of the values and beliefs, but more detailing is needed for the theory itself to become more holistic. Ethical knowing in relation to ethical theories, principles and codes are distinctly referred to. Healthcare professionals are expected to provide care with an ethically acute and sensitive attitude (Shaha, 2014: 138). The importance of collaboration within the interprofessional healthcare team are explicitly mentioned. Collaboration and nurturance as specified by Bergum (1994) are evident. Further detailing through research is needed regarding adequate interventions to promote interprofessional collaboration.

The theory not only includes aspects that are important for implementation in practice, but also provides insight into ethical knowing. Issues such as existentiality, spirituality, end-of-life questions and related ethical topics are mentioned as part of the theory (Shaha, 2014). Hence healthcare professionals need to develop ethical knowing to propose adequate interventions to patients and their families. Healthcare professionals are expected to listen to the patients' narrative and the families' concerns and, in response, be attentive to possibly confusing or incomplete information being provided.

Case example for practice

A 65-year-old woman, married, with two adult children living on their own and owning a farm together with her husband (also over 65 years), is considered in this case example. The husband is still farming (livestock and arable crops) with a large household. The woman has a stage 4 colorectal cancer and undergone surgery. She has received a temporary colostomy. The patient does not have much pain, but has to undergo radiotherapy and chemotherapy treatments. She worries as she lives about 25 km away from the hospital and public transport is limited due to the rural area in which she and her husband live. Therefore, she will have to rely on the husband's help and on a neighbour for support.

Treatment is advancing well. The temporary colostomy presents a minor problem. The patient is looking forward to completing her treatments and having the colostomy closed. Her healthcare professionals have confirmed that the treatment will end in two weeks. Hence, reversing the colostomy will happen in another four weeks.

At the next consultation and treatment, where the husband is present, the woman is told by the physician that the colostomy needs to remain in situ for an additional two months, as the cancer treatment must be prolonged to improve the outcome of the disease. International recommendations had recently changed, therefore to reduce the risk of recurrence, the prolongation is recommended. The woman and her husband are shocked and dismayed as their hopes to finish treatment as planned fall apart and the couple argue determinately against it. For the healthcare professionals, their decision making is considered difficult because of the recommendations for good practice are the extension of the treatment and postponing the closure of the colostomy. In the subsequent discussion, the nurse encourages the woman and her husband to state their fears, concerns and wishes openly and clearly (care ethics; narrative ethics). The nurse particularly encourages the woman and her husband to tell their story of the limitations they have encountered since the diagnosis. The woman and her husband also explain that the closure of the colostomy is important for them (autonomy) as they will be attending their daughter's wedding, which was planned to coincide with the time schedule given earlier. Knowing of the new treatment recommendations (beneficence) and supporting the physician's intention to do good (virtue ethics) and the couple's need also to control the situation (feminist ethics), the nurse judges that a compromise could be struck. In consideration of the theory *The Omnipresence of Cancer*, the nurse aims at transparency and at highlighting the benefits and drawbacks for each of the actors, including herself. Together, they decide that instead of waiting two months, but rather waiting only one month is possible before the colostomy is closed, with both sides gaining what they wanted and assuming responsibility for the extra giving and taking.

Conclusion

Selecting a theory for practice is influenced by the selectors' values, beliefs and attitudes. It is therefore necessary to identify these elements in a theory. Based on these findings, the theory's acceptability by the healthcare professionals and the clinical practice where it is supposed to be used, can be determined. Uncovering the basic values and beliefs of a theory will help to identify the information on caring described by Roach (2002) and Tronto (1993). Hence, it is possible to create an ethically sensitive practice and provide such care to patients and their families. Caring can then be negotiated in the clinical area and relevant and adequate interventions can be identified, developed and implemented in respective clinical practice.

The theory of *The Omnipresence of Cancer* focuses on patients with life-threatening diseases and offers additional understanding. This theory requires nurses to be caring in the way described by Roach (2002) and Tronto (1993), to exercise ethical knowing and provide holistic and ethical care to patients.

Specific practice for different groups of healthcare professionals can be identified with the help of the theory, i.e., advanced nursing care, spiritual care and supportive care. A number of aspects of ethical knowing have been described explicitly in the theory. To improve usefulness and implementation in practice, further clarification is needed through research. In addition, further exploration of the contribution of ethical knowing to the theory is necessary. Implementation of the theory into practice is important to determine impact on patient outcomes.

Appendix

Table 5.7 Theory analysis and evaluation by McEwen and Wills (2007: 109) and the theory analysis by Smith and Parker (2015: 21–22)

McEwen and Wills (2007: 109)	Smith and Parker (2015: 21–22)
1. Theory description	1. How is nursing conceptualized in the theory?
• What is the purpose of the theory? (describe, explain, predict, prescribe) • What is the scope or level of the theory? (grand, middle range, practice) • What are the origins of the theory? • What are the major concepts? • What are the major theoretical propositions? • What are the major assumptions? • Is the context for use described?	Is the focus of nursing stated? • What does the nurse attend to when practicing nursing? • What guides nursing observations, reflections, decisions, and actions? • What illustrations or examples show how the theory is used to guide practice? What is the purpose of nursing? • What do nurses do when they are practicing nursing based on the theory? • What are the examples of nursing assessment, designs, plans, and evaluations? • What indicators give evidence of the quality of nursing practice? • Is the richness and complexity of nursing practice evident?

(Continued)

Table 5.7 (Continued)

McEwen and Wills (2007: 109)	Smith and Parker (2015: 21–22)
	What are the boundaries or limits for nursing? • How is nursing distinguished from other health-related professions? • How is nursing related to other disciplines and services? • What is the place of nursing in interprofessional practice? • What is the range of nursing situations in which the theory is useful? How can nursing situations be described? • What are the attributes of the recipient of nursing care? • What are the characteristics of the nurse? • Are there environmental requirements for the practice of nursing? If so, what are they?
2. Theory analysis • Are concepts theoretically and operationally defined? • Are statements theoretically and operationally defined? • Are linkages explicit? • Is the theory logically organized? • Is there a model/diagram? Does the model contribute to clarifying the theory? • Are concepts, statements and assumptions used consistently? • Are the outcomes or consequences stated or predicted?	2. What is the context of the theory development? Who is the nursing theorist as person and as nurse? • Why did the theorist develop the theory? • What is the background of the theorist as a nursing scholar? • What central values and beliefs does the theorist set forth? What are the major theoretical influences on this theory? • What previous knowledge influenced the development of this theory? • What are the relationships between this theory and other theories? • What nursing-related theories and philosophies influenced this theory? What were major external influences on development of the theory? • What were the social, economic, and political influences that informed the theory? • What images of nurses and nursing influenced the development of the theory? • What was the status of nursing as s discipline and profession at the time of the theory's development?
3. Theory evaluation • Is the theory congruent with current nursing standards? • Is the theory congruent with current nursing interventions or therapeutics? • Has the theory been tested empirically? Is it supported by research? Does it appear to be accurate/valid?	3. Who are authoritative sources for information about development, evaluation, and use of this theory? Which nursing authorities speak about, write about, and use the theory? • What are the professional attributes of these persons? • What are the attributes of authorities, and how does one become one? • Which others can be considered authorities?

• Is there evidence that the theory has been used by nursing educators, nursing researchers, or nursing administrators? • Is the theory socially relevant? • Is the theory relevant cross-culturally? • Does the theory contribute to the discipline of nursing? • What are the implications for nursing related to implementation of the theory?	What major resources are authoritative sources on the theory? • What books, articles, and audiovisual and electronic media exist to elucidate the theory? • What nursing organizations share and support work related to the theory? • What service and academic programs are authoritative sources for practicing and teaching the theory?

4. How can the overall significance of the nursing theory be described?

What is the importance of the nursing theory over time?
• What are exemplars of the theory's use that structure and guide individual practice?
• How has the theory been used to guide programs of nursing education?
• How has the theory been used to guide nursing administration and organizations?
• How does published nursing scholarship reflect the significance of the theory?

What is the experience of nurses who report consistent use of the theory?
• What is the range of reports from practice?
• Has nursing research led to further theoretical formulations?
• Has the theory been used to develop new nursing practices?
• Has the theory influenced the design of methods of nursing inquiry?
• What has been the influence of the theory on nursing and health policy?

What are the projected influences of the theory on nursing's future?
• How has the theory influenced the community of scholars?
• In what ways has nursing as a professional practice been strengthened by the theory?
• What future possibilities for nursing have been opened because of this theory?
• What will be the continuing social value of the theory?

Legend: Among others, McEwen and Wills (2007) and Smith and Parker (2015) propose questions and guidance for analysing and/or evaluating nursing theory. McEwen and Wills (2007) have reviewed the propositions by various authors. Adapted from these suggestions, McEwen and Wills (2007: 109) developed their own theory analysis and evaluation. In contrast, Smith and Parker (2015) focus on the relevance and possibility of implementation of nursing theory into practice. Hence, the questions proposed by Smith and Parker (2015: 21–22) focus predominantly on practice relevance. The criteria stated above can be used to analyse a theory. For evaluation of the theory, Smith and Parker (2015) propose to consider the existing sets of criteria in relation to the scope of the theory.

Notes

1 In nursing, the term 'theory' is often understood as part of a ladder of abstraction (Fawcett and Desanto-Madeya, 2013). A more abstract form of nursing knowledge is the conceptual model, which involves a number of concepts that are connected to one another through assumptions and propositions. Theories can also be on different levels of abstraction, ranging from large to micro theories. In this chapter, the term 'theory' is used to denote all of these forms of knowledge to facilitate reading.
2 For the whole list of questions that Smith, M. C. and Parker, M. E. 2015. *Nursing Theories and Nursing Practice*. Philadelphia, PA: F. A. Davis. propose for theory analysis, see the Appendix.

References

Armstrong, A. E. 2006. Towards a strong virtue ethics for nursing practice. *Nursing Philosophy*, 7, 110–24.

Beauchamp, T. L. and Childress, J. F. 1979. *Principles of Biomedical Ethics*. New York: Oxford University Press.

Beauchamp, T. L. and Childress, J. F. 2013. *Principles of Biomedical Ethics*. New York: Oxford University Press.

Benner, P. E. 2001. *From Novice to Expert: Excellence and Power in Clinical Nursing Practice*. Upper Saddle River, NJ: Prentice Hall.

Bergum, V. 1994. Knowledge for ethical care. *Nursing Ethics*, 1, 71–9.

Carper, B. 1978. Fundamental patterns of knowing in nursing. *ANS. Advances in Nursing Science*, 1, 13–23.

Chinn, P. L. and Kramer, M. K. 2015. *Knowledge Development in Nursing: Theory and Process*. St. Louis, MO: Elsevier Mosby.

Da Rocha, M. G., Roos, P. and Shaha, M. 2014. Le sentiment de finitude de vie et les stratégies de coping face à l'annonce d'un cancer. *Revue internationale de soins palliatifs*, 29, 49–53.

De Raeve, L. 2006. Virtue ethics. In A. J. Davis, L. De Raeve and V. Tschudin (eds.), *Essentials of Teaching and Learning in Nursing Ethics: Perspectives and Methods*. Edinburgh: Churchill Livingstone.

Degrazia, D. and Brand-Ballard, J. 2011. *Biomedical Ethics*. New York: McGraw-Hill Higher Education.

Dubose, E. R., Hamel, R. P. and O'Connell, L. J. 1994. *A Matter of Principles?: Ferment in U.S. Bioethics*. Valley Forge, PA: Trinity Press International.

Fawcett, J. and Desanto-Madeya, S. 2013. *Contempory Nursing Knowledge: Analysis and Evaluation of Nursing Models and Theories*. Philadelphia, PA: F.A. Davis.

Frank, A. 1954. *The Diary of a Young Girl*. Vallentine: Mitchell.

Gaillard Desmedt, S. and Shaha, M. 2013. Le rôle de la spiritualité dans les soins infirmiers: une revue de littérature. *Recherche en soins infirmiers*, 115, 19–35.

Gastmans, C. 2006. The care perspective in healthcare ethics. In A. J. Davis, L. De Raeve and V. Tschudin (eds.), *Essentials of Teaching and Learning in Nursing Ethics: Perspectives and Methods*. Edinburgh: Churchill Livingstone.

Gilligan, C. 1982. *In a Different Voice: Psychological Theory and Women's Development*. Cambridge, MA; London: Harvard University Press.

Grace, P. J. and Milliken, A. 2016. Educating nurses for ethical practice in contemporary health care environments. *Hastings Center Report*, 46(Suppl 1), S13–7.

Held, V. 2006. *The Ethics of Care: Personal, Political, and Global.* Oxford; New York: Oxford University Press.

Institute of Medicine. 2010. The future of nursing. Leading change, advancing health. *Advising the Nation/Improving Health* [Online].

Institute of Medicine. 2013. *Delivering High-Quality Cancer Care*, ed. by Institute of Medicine. Washington: IOM.

Kant, I. 1986. *Grundlegung zur Metaphysik der Sitten.* Ditzingen: Reclam.

Kohlberg, L. 1981. *The Philosophy of Moral Development: Moral Stages and the Idea of Justice.* San Francisco; London: Harper & Row.

Liaschenko, J. and Peter, E. 2003. Feminist ethics. In V. Tschudin (ed.), *Approaches to Ethics: Nursing Beyond Boundaries.* Edinburgh: Butterworth-Heinemann.

Maslow, A. H. 1970. *Motivation and Personality*, second edition. New York; London: Harper & Row.

McEwen, M. and Wills, E. M. 2007. *Theoretical Basis for Nursing.* Philadelphia, PA: Lippincott Williams & Wilkins.

McKenna, H. P., Pajnkihar, M. and Murphy, F. 2015. *Fundamentals of Nursing Models, Theories and Practice.* Wiley-Blackwell.

Murdoch, I. 1970. *The Sovereignty of Good.* London: Routledge, 1991.

Niebuhr, H. R. 1963. *The Responsible Self. An Essay in Christian Moral Philosophy.* With an introduction by James M. Gustafson. New York: Harper & Row.

Nightingale, F. 1879. *Letter From Florence Nightingale to the Probationer-Nurses in the "Nightingale Fund" School at St. Thomas' Hospital: Easter, 1879*, [S.l.: s.n.].

Noddings, N. 1984. *Caring: A Feminine Approach to Ethics and Moral Education.* Berkeley: University of California Press, c1984 (1986).

O'Neill, O. 1991. Introducing ethics: some current positions. *Bulletin of Medical Ethics*, 73, 18–21.

Roach, M. S. 1984. *Caring: The Human Mode of Being, Implications for Nursing.* Toronto: University of Toronto, Faculty of Nursing.

Roach, M. S. 2002. *The Human Act of Caring: A Blueprint for the Health Professions.* Ottawa: Canadian Hospital Association Press, c1992 (1999 [printing]).

Shaha, M. 2003. Life with intestinal cancer. A phenomenologic-empirical study. *Pflege*, 16, 323–30.

Shaha, M. 2014. The omnipresence of cancer. In From The Chair of Family Orientated and Community Nursing, F. O. H., Department of Nursing Science (ed.), *Cumulative Thesis in Partial Fulfilment of Obtaining the Venia Legendi for the Subject of Nursing Science of the Faculty of Health, Department of Nursing Science of the University Witten/ Herdecke.* Witten/Herdecke, Germany: University of Witten/Herdecke.

Shaha, M. and Bauer-Wu, S. 2009. Early adulthood uprooted: transitoriness in young women with breast cancer. *Cancer Nursing*, 32, 246–55.

Shaha, M. and Cox, C. L. 2003. The omnipresence of cancer. *European Journal of Oncology Nursing*, 7, 191–6.

Shaha, M., Cox, C. L., Belcher, A. E. and Cohen, M. Z. 2011. Transitoriness: patients' perception of life after a diagnosis of cancer. *Cancer Nursing Practice*, 10, 24–7.

Shaha, M., Cox, C. L., Hall, A., Porrett, T. and Brown, J. 2006. The omnipresence of cancer: its implications for colorectal cancer. *Cancer Nursing Practice*, 5, 35–9.

Shaha, M., Cox, C. L., Talman, K. and Kelly, D. 2008. Uncertainty in breast, prostate, and colorectal cancer: implications for supportive care. *Journal of Nursing Scholarship*, 40, 60–7.

Shaha, M., Pandian, V., Choti, M. A., Stotsky, E., Herman, J. M., Khan, Y., Libonati, C., Pawlik, T. M., Schulick, R. D. and Belcher, A. E. 2010. Transitoriness in cancer patients:

a cross-sectional survey of lung and gastrointestinal cancer patients. *Supportive Care in Cancer*, 19, 271–9.

Smith, M. C. and Parker, M. E. 2015. *Nursing Theories and Nursing Practice*. Philadelphia, PA: F. A. Davis.

Tronto, J. C. 1993. *Moral Boundaries: A Political Argument for an Ethic of Care*. New York; London: Routledge.

Tschudin, V. 1999. *Nurses Matter: Reclaiming Our Professional Identity*. Basingstoke: Macmillan.

Tschudin, V. 2003a. *Approaches to Ethics: Nursing Beyond Boundaries*. Edinburgh: Butterworth-Heinemann.

Tschudin, V. 2003b. *Ethics in Nursing: The Caring Relationship*. Edinburgh: Butterworth-Heinemann.

White, J. 1995. Patterns of knowing: review, critique, and update. *ANS. Advances in Nursing Science*, 17, 73–86.

6 Transitoriness

Instrument development

M. Zumstein-Shaha and G. T. Sobral

Introduction

Despite scientific progress in the field of Oncology, a cancer diagnosis remains associated with death. Patients experience a sense of the finitude of life, which is called Transitoriness by Shaha (Shaha, 2003; Shaha and Cox, 2003; Borges et al., 2006). At this moment, patients are confronted with thoughts of their own death. One's own demise becomes a reality the moment a cancer diagnosis is made. The experience of life's finitude and confrontation with death is also present within the patient's circle of acquaintances and healthcare professionals associated with Oncology (de Oliveira et al., 2013; Junior et al., 2011).

In recent years, advances in diagnostics, treatment and medical devices in Oncology have contributed to increased life expectancy and recovery rates, but also a greater complexity of care (Howard-Anderson et al., 2012). Modern medicine has predominantly focused on biological or related aspects of the cancer disease at the expense of social, cultural and psychological aspects (Shaha et al., 2011a; Woodgate et al., 2014; Sjovall et al., 2011). To date, special attention is needed to conceptualize the disease experience of patients (Sjovall et al., 2011; Woodgate et al., 2014; Lehto and Stein, 2009). Psychosocial needs are assessed by healthcare professionals. However, enforcement of psychosocial needs and suitable interventions continues to be defective. Low application rates in care practices are seen, as well as a lack of institutional guidelines and policies (Surbone et al., 2010). An understanding of the existential impact of cancer remains unknown. *The Omnipresence of Cancer* (Shaha, 2003; Shaha, 2014; Shaha and Cox, 2003; Shaha, 2016b) as a theory, represents a possible solution.

Transitoriness is one of three concepts present within the dimension of "Toward Authentic Dasein". Toward Authentic Dasein is one of the two main constructs in the theory *The Omnipresence of Cancer* (Shaha, 2003). The concept termed Transitoriness documents the experience of the finitude of life resulting from the impact of living with and fighting cancer (Shaha et al., 2006). After conducting a concept analysis of Transitoriness, a preliminary instrument has been developed to provide professionals with a tool that can be used at different stages of the cancer disease (Cox et al., 2012; Shaha et al., 2011b) to identify the perceptions patients have of Transitoriness so that better care can be provided. The goal of nursing related to Transitoriness is the support of patients in their experience of the finitude of life and managing this experience.

This chapter initially describes the concept of Transitoriness and the nursing care associated with this concept. This is followed by explicating the development of a preliminary instrument according to the methodology of DeVellis (2012). The process of content validation and pre-test of the instrument will be discussed (DeVellis, 2012; Polit et al., 2007). The methodologies of content validation and pre-testing of the Transitoriness instrument will be included. Validation results as well as the pre-test results will be presented.

Transitoriness

In cancer, patients experience several moments of grief due to diagnosis of the life-threatening disease and its subsequent treatments (Dolina et al., 2013). Patients experience anxiety, uncertainty and depression, which are associated with fear of death and the non-achievement of some of their objectives in life. In order to deal with the disease, patients seek to give meaning to the diagnosis, to redefine the future, to manage daily life and continue to be themselves (Dunn et al., 2006). Finitude of life is no longer a futile thought, it becomes a real possibility. Patients are in an ambivalent situation; having to conceptualize the finiteness of life, while looking forward into the future (Shaha et al., 2011a). Although these experiences are opposite, they are negatively associated with one another. Managing the disease is impacted by these two opposite experiences (Tang et al., 2011). Questions about death, about the meaning of life and one's beliefs arise (Dolina et al., 2013; Woodgate et al., 2014). A confrontation with death is often associated with feelings of loneliness, the feeling of being disconnected from one's surroundings and living a unique experience (Shaha, 2003; Bouché and Bernhard, 2011). Patients also suffer a decline in quality of life associated with the disease (Dolina et al., 2013).

The concept of Transitoriness consists of three attributes: awareness of the threatened life, anxiety, and change. Awareness of the threatened life is manifested by a feeling that life is transient due to the perception of cancer being a life-threatening disease. As a response to this threat, patients experience a fear of death in general and the subsequent circumstances of their own death. This first attribute (awareness of the threatened life) is also related to the preparation of one's own death, the funeral and the formulation of farewells. In practice, patients may decide to put their affairs in order, to consider leaving a legacy and/ or to reunite their family members (Shaha et al., 2011a; Shaha and Bauer-Wu, 2009; Shaha et al., 2010). The second attribute, anxiety, is based on fear of death, which can provoke feelings of distress and uncertainty. Aspects of the disease and treatments elicit uncertainty, which can lead to loss of autonomy or loss of control (Shaha and Bauer-Wu, 2009). The attribute of change includes elements of novelty and standardization. As a result of becoming aware of the threat to one's life and through the experience of anxiety, patients redefine or conceptualize new values. In addition, one's perception of self as well as relationships with family members or other persons may change. Patients then move into a new phase of life that can be called standardization or normalization. As part of this phase, patients integrate the disease into their daily lives (Shaha and Bauer-Wu, 2009; Shaha et al., 2011a). Transitoriness, as a concept, is fully developed within the theory *The Omnipresence of Cancer* (Shaha, 2003; Shaha and Cox, 2003).

Background

The concept of Transitoriness

The theory of *The Omnipresence of Cancer* incorporates the concept Transitoriness. This concept described the experience of being confronted with life's finitude following a cancer diagnosis. This experience of the finiteness of life had been described previously (Little and Sayers, 2004b; Little and Sayers, 2004a; Cohen et al., 2004), but had not yet been fully described or conceptualized as part of a theory. Therefore, no adequate instrument to assess this experience existed. In addition, this experience was often subsumed within the concept of "fear of death" or "death awareness" (Cohen et al., 2004; Shaha et al., 2010). Due to a lack of adequate measurements, various instruments were used to assess Transitoriness in the early works by Shaha et al. (Shaha et al., 2010). For example, the State-Trait Personality Inventory by Spielberger had been employed (Shaha et al., 2010). These early works demonstrated that the experience of Transitoriness played an important role in cancer patients' trajectories (Shaha and Bauer-Wu, 2009; Shaha et al., 2010). However, the instruments used in these early works predominantly assessed only one or two aspects of the experience of life's finitude. They did not evaluate Transitoriness in its entirety. As a result, Shaha et al. (Shaha et al., 2006) conducted an evolutionary concept analysis of Transitoriness. A total of three attributes were identified. These are awareness of life's finitude, anxiety and change. Table 6.1 provides a description of the attributes of Transitoriness.

Morse et al. have identified several criteria for identifying a concept and also determine its degree of maturity (Morse et al., 1996). These are shown in Table 6.2.

Drawing on Morse et al. (Morse et al., 1996), the concept of Transitoriness has been defined (Shaha et al., 2006). To date, no conflicting definition is being used. Transitoriness is defined as: "the experience of transitoriness is a reaction to a cancer diagnosis, the difficulty envisioning a future and subsequent adjustment to the realization of life's transitory nature" (Shaha et al., 2011a: 26).

Table 6.1 Attributes of the concept of Transitoriness

Dimension	Sub-categories	Description
Awareness of life's finitude	• Threat to life • Thoughts of death • Leaving the world behind	Patients become aware of their life, their situation, and their remaining time (Adelbratt and Strang, 2000; Winterling et al., 2004)
Anxiety	• Fear • Distress • Uncertainty	Patients fear dying and wrestle with the thought of death (Barroilhet Diez et al., 2005; Blinderman and Cherny, 2005; Esbensen et al., 2008).
Change	• New • Self • Relationships • Normalization	Patients have a chance to reassess and/or conceptualize new values (Adelbratt and Strang, 2000; Barroilhet Diez et al., 2005)

Legend: This table is adapted from Shaha et al. (Shaha et al., 2011a: 25).

Table 6.2 Criteria for concept evaluation

	Indices of concept maturity	
Criteria	Emerging	Mature
Concept definition	Lacks clarity Competing definitions	Clear Consensual
Characteristics	Not identified	Clearly described
Preconditions and outcomes	Not identified	Described fully and demonstrated
Boundaries	Not known	Delineated

Legend: This table is adapted from Morse et al. (Morse et al., 1996).

When considering the nature of Transitoriness, it has been found that similar concepts have been identified, namely "death anxiety", "death awareness", "death salience", "mortality salience" and "liminality". The concept of "hope" constitutes a contrary concept. An antecedent for the concept of Transitoriness is the diagnosis of a life-threatening disease such as cancer (Shaha et al., 2006). In view of the aforementioned, it can be concluded that the concept of Transitoriness has obtained maturity. However, concepts are subject to changes over time; therefore, further research will be necessary as time passes.

The development of the concept of Transitoriness contributes to the advancement of the theory, *The Omnipresence of Cancer*. Transitoriness as a concept promotes documentation of patients' experiences of being diagnosed with cancer. To date, a paucity of research exists in relation to this experience. Some studies are being conducted in fulfillment of Master's of Science in Nursing and Doctoral Programmes in Nursing Science. These studies use the theory, *The*

Omnipresence of Cancer as a frame of reference for the research. Most of the studies are being conducted in the French-speaking part of Switzerland. Hence, healthcare professionals practicing in this part of Switzerland are familiar with the theory and the concept of Transitoriness. Having been educated about this theory through research conducted in practice, healthcare professionals have had the opportunity to become aware of related works, research methodologies and subsequently developed a way of working with students while the students are undertaking their research. As a result, healthcare professionals are participating closely in the advancement of the theory. It is evident there is a link that has been created between the practice environment and academic setting; promoting future works. One of the primary areas of research related to the concept (Transitoriness), is development of an instrument (sometimes termed an Inventory) for the purpose of furthering knowledge associated with the theory *The Omnipresence of Cancer.*

The development process

Several steps are required for the psychometric development of a valid and reliable instrument. DeVellis (2012) recommends eight steps. The objective of DeVellis (2012) methodology is to provide a guideline for developing instruments (DeVellis, 2012). These steps are: a) Generation of an item pool, b) Determination of the response type of the instrument, c) Expert consultation on the Item pool, d) Integration of the expert consultation, e) Item administration to the target population, f) Determination of item assessment and g) Scale optimization.

Generating an item pool

Items are developed based on a theoretical basis or on existing research (DeVellis, 2012; Rust and Golombok, 2015). For the development of an instrument of Transitoriness, the items were generated based on the concept analysis undertaken by Shaha et al. (2011a).

Determination of the response type of the instrument

Various formats of evaluating responses exist. For example, instruments can be divided into norm-reference or criterion-referenced measures. The norm-reference measures help assess one person's performance against the performance of persons in a similar group, whereas criterion-reference measures help assess a person's performance against a pre-determined set of criteria that is developed in conjunction with the preliminary instrument. Both types of instruments require validation in a target population. However, depending on the type of instrument, different response formats apply (Waltz et al., 2010). The preliminary instrument of Transitoriness falls into the first type of instrument, i.e., the norm-reference measures. As such, various response formats such as yes or no answers or Likert-type scales can be employed (Waltz et al., 2010). Likert scales are fairly common. Such response formats deliver ordinal data. It is recommended to utilize five-point Likert scales or two more response points or two less (i.e., three to seven response options for a Likert scale) on an instrument. Response options greater than seven are considered an overload (Streiner et al., 2008; McDowell, 2006). The numbers associated with the response options of a Likert scale are arbitrary (McDowell, 2006). However, numbers from 1 to 5 are fairly common (Streiner et al., 2008; McDowell, 2006).

Expert consultation on the item pool

An important step in the process of instrument development is feedback obtained in expert consultations. It is recommended the researcher identify experts within the field of the theme that should be explored by the future instrument as well as experts from practice (DeVellis, 2012; Waltz et al., 2010).

Integration of expert consultation

For integrating the experts' recommendations, the item content validity index (I-CVI) is calculated. The I-CVI is an alternative to the more current content validity index (CVI). The I-CVI evaluates the relevance of each item using a four point Likert scale ranging from irrelevant to very relevant. More specifically, an I-CVI adjusted to the probability of chance that the item is evaluated relevant or irrelevant is used for the instrument of Transitoriness. For each item, the number of quotations equal to three and four is added and then divided by the number of experts. An I-CVI greater than 0.72 is necessary in order to validate the item (Polit, Beck and Owen, 2007). The validation of content is a critical and vital process to establish measurement reliability. It concerns the degree of relevance of each item to represent the phenomenon of interest (Waltz et al., 2010). Experts are expected to evaluate the degree to which the preliminary instrument represents the phenomenon of interest (Fortin and Gagnon, 2010). The preliminary instrument that is submitted to the experts includes the purpose of the instrument and information about the phenomenon of interest as it is represented on/in a theoretical basis. If a preliminary instrument consists of sub-dimensions (such as is the case with Transitoriness), the definitions of these sub-dimensions are provided for the convenience of the experts with the four point Likert scale for the evaluation and for calculation of the I-CVI. In addition, experts can be asked to comment on their reasons for attributing a judgment of "not relevant or irrelevant".

Item administration to the target population

Subsequent, to integration of the experts' recommendations, and the calculation of the I-CVI, the preliminary instrument is ready to be administered to the target population. At this point, the approval of a local ethics committee must be obtained.

Determination of item assessment (scale optimization)

This last step requires the renewed administration of the preliminary instrument within the target population. However, this time, a total of 5–10 responses per item need to be obtained. Subsequently, statistical analyses are conducted to test the scale structure (Waltz et al., 2010; McDowell, 2006; Streiner et al., 2008). Based on the statistical tests, it is possible to determine whether the instrument consists of subscales and specific information on the analysis of the instrument can be determined.

Discussion

The instrument of Transitoriness

Use of DeVellis's (2012) method, within the context of the development of the Transitoriness instrument, has allowed a constant evolution as well as its evaluation through various samplings. This chapter highlights the results achieved during the validation stages of content and pre-test of the instrument. The first phase involved a focus on elderly patients with chronic disease. The second involved a focus on patients with cancer.

Generating an item pool

The concept analysis of Transitoriness (Shaha et al., 2011b) provided a sound basis for the generation of items for the instrument. Two rounds for discerning items were conducted.

PRELIMINARY ITEMS

Firstly, questions in English were constructed based on the descriptions of the attributes of Transitoriness. These questions could either be responded to by

Table 6.3 The structure of the preliminary instrument of Transitoriness

Description of the dimension	
Formulation of items	Desired response format

Legend: For each dimension, items were formulated according to the concept analysis (Shaha et al., 2011b).

using a Likert rating scale or yes and no. A total of 51 items were compiled that were arranged into the attributes of Transitoriness. This list of questions was submitted to a group of three experts. All experts were nurse scholars, native English speakers, who reside in the United Kingdom and the United States. Some editing recommendations were made, but otherwise the questions were considered acceptable to be administered to patients. An I-CUI was not calculated at this juncture. Therefore, this preliminary instrument did not possess any psychometric properties. At this stage, the instrument resembled a survey, which was used in a Master's thesis (Pantic, 2015). After forward-backward translation into Italian (Wild et al., 2005), the survey was administered to elderly persons suffering from chronic diseases such as heart failure and COPD. Besides the preliminary instrument, the study participants were asked to complete an instrument measuring their evaluation of proximity to death. Despite the survey-character of the preliminary instrument, some interesting associations were found. Elderly patients with chronic diseases experience thoughts of death, are not really fearful or anxious about it and do not envision changes due to their life-threatening disease. These patients are aware of their proximity to death. This is accepted as part of their daily life. The participants in Pantic's study (Pantic, 2015) emphasized that thoughts of death or thinking about the proximity of their own death were daily occurrences and were not necessarily stressful. Experiencing and managing the finitude of life were considered important topics. Hence, it was determined feasible to submit instruments with such questions to people with chronic diseases.

FINAL ITEM POOL

In order to develop a psychometrically sound instrument, the list of items was extended from the first 51 items to a total of 79 items. At this time, the items were translated into French, and additional items were added for testing. These items were arranged per attribute of Transitoriness, i.e., consciousness, anxiety and change. The following table summarizes the structure:

The items were classified in chronological order of the attributes of the concept of Transitoriness. To each of the attributes, subcategories were added, namely: 1) Being aware of the disease; 2) Thoughts related to death; 3) Thoughts other than sadness related to death and 4) Living with changes.

Determination of the response format

It was decided that a five-point Likert scale should serve as the response format. The response options ranged from "quite agree" to "strongly disagree". As not all items allowed for a response on a five-point Likert scale, all 79 items were reviewed and reformulated where necessary. Item construction was directed toward stating items in a positive manner. Thus, an important step in producing a psychometrically sound instrument was achieved.

Expert consultation on the item pool and integration of the comments

For the purpose of further development of the instrument a second research project was undertaken. In this project, experts were selected from the field of nursing practice and scholarship, medical ethics, theology, psycho-oncology and medicine. This time the instrument was developed in French; therefore, all experts who formed the review panel were native French speakers. The panel of 11 experts was considered to be experts in the care of newly diagnosed cancer patients. A total of seven participants had a nursing background; three experts were physicians, and one expert was psychologist. Of these experts, four practiced in research settings.

A total of three rounds of soliciting experts were conducted. During the first round, experts were asked to consider each item for its suitability and its formulation. The experts were also asked to consider the items in relation to the descriptions of the concept of Transitoriness and its dimensions. Based on the experts' responses, the I-CVI was calculated. At the end of two rounds, the number of items on the instrument was reduced from 79 to 46. Of these 46 items, 74% obtained an excellent I-CVI with ratings between 0.90 and 1; whereas 26% achieved an acceptable I-CVI around 0.72 (Polit et al., 2007). All comments by the experts were considered and analyzed. Following the aforementioned, a third round was conducted. The purpose of this round was to obtain an agreement on the feasibility of administering the preliminary instrument to the target patient group. A third round is not usually included in expert consultations. However, it was decided to have a third round as the topic of the preliminary instrument is sensitive and can potentially unsettle a respondent.

Finally, the preliminary instrument was submitted to clinical nurse specialists of the collaborating department of care where it would be administered to patients. Between each round of consultations, the preliminary instrument's content and wording were reviewed. Thus, the content of the preliminary instrument evolved into a more comprehensible format. As previously indicated, it is important to understand that having the third round of expert consultation and submitting the preliminary instrument to nurses with a clinical specialist background do not constitute essential steps of the validation process (Polit and Beck, 2010; Polit et al., 2007). However, these two adjustments were made in the light of the sensitivity of the instrument's topic and the risk of unsettling the target population. Furthermore, the additional steps helped to prepare the approach to the target population, to answer the questions of healthcare professionals, and to promote integration of the research into the clinical setting. From these last steps, the final version of the preliminary instrument emerged. It was then used for the pre-test in target population. In this final version, the preliminary instrument was extended to include an

Table 6.4 Format of the instrument of Transitoriness

Since my cancer diagnosis . . .					
I am able to manage my disease	Fully agree	Totally agree	Agree	Do not agree	Strongly disagree
I fear uncontrollable symptoms	Fully agree	Totally agree	Agree	Do not agree	Strongly disagree

Legend: Part of narrative on the instrument of Transitoriness prior to submission to the experts.

introductory note. A few sentences were added to explain the purpose of the instrument and to provide explanatory instructions. Patients responding to the instrument were led into the questions by the sentence: "Since my cancer diagnosis". All items are formulated in an affirmative response that can be qualified by a five point Likert scale. The respondent is invited to circle the respective answer. Table 6.4 provides an example of questions (statements) on the instrument (Inventory).

In the final version of the instrument, items regarding end of life and death are situated in the middle of the instrument. At the beginning and at the end, questions about the current health situation and potential changes in life are stated. Thus, the instrument does not start with potentially sensitive questions. The items were categorized according to the three dimensions of the instrument, which enable analysis as recommended by Tavares (2015).

Item administration to the target population

During pre-test of the instrument, comprehension of the items and reception of the sensitive topic were explored with the target population. The pretest involved administering the instrument of Transitoriness followed by a cognitive interview. The cognitive interview was semi-directed (involved semi-structured questions). In the interview, the following four aspects were explored: patients' reactions following administration of the instrument, formulation of the items and link with the dimension, evaluation of the clarity of the instrument and patients' comments concerning the Likert scale.

The pre-testing process involved two rounds of pilot testing the preliminary instrument. In each round, a total of n = 10 patients were included. Therefore, a total of n = 20 patients diagnosed with cancer between six months and one year participated in the pre-test. All participants were receiving medical treatment. Between each round, the instrument was revised. Feedback and comments made by the participants were integrated into the instrument (Inventory). The results provided data that were both quantitative and qualitative. Qualitative data were obtained as previously mentioned through semi-directed interviews.

In addition to the preliminary instrument of Transitoriness being administered, participants were asked to complete a questionnaire about sociodemographic data such as age or gender. The sociodemographic questionnaires completed by the participants were analyzed with descriptive statistics and correlations. The findings offer a preliminary overview of trends and relationships between the three dimensions (consciousness, anxiety, change) of the instrument of Transitoriness as well as with the patients' sociodemographic data.

Completing the preliminary instrument of Transitoriness determined that it does not cause emotional distress when participants complete the instrument. There is no change between completing the questionnaire and five days post-completion. However, it was found that items that included the term "death" were considered to be too direct by four patients. Nevertheless, these four patients did not have any negative reactions following completion of the instrument. Participants consider the preliminary instrument to be reflective of their disease and treatment experience. Comprehension of the items was considered good. Nevertheless, the five-point Likert scale was considered too detailed by three participants and too crude by two other participants. These findings indicated a need to further refine the instrument.

Overall, participants reacted positively to administration of the instrument. In conclusion, participants considered the instrument applicable to their disease and treatment experience. Their responses reflected those of the experts who were consulted during the validation process.

Nursing care

Patients' experiences of Transitoriness necessitate nursing care based on an understanding of *The Omnipresence of Cancer* as a theory in association with its concept Transitoriness. Patients' conceptualization of the experience of cancer and the meaning attributed to the disease require addressing by nurses administering nursing care to this group (Shaha et al., 2006). The goal of nursing care when patients experience Transitoriness is to help them understand their diagnosis and prognosis and sense of finitude of life that subsequently ensues. This element of nursing care is essential so that patients can adapt to changes in their everyday lives in association with its treatment modalities (Shaha et al., 2011a). Addressing the experience of Transitoriness will help patients begin to regain control as well as "map out" their future (Shaha et al., 2006; Shaha et al., 2010; Shaha et al., 2011b) .

Nursing care in relation to the concept Transitoriness includes a systematic assessment of the impact of cancer on patients' lives and assisting them to confront the finitude of life, as well as their long-term follow-up throughout the patients' continuum of care. Drawing on this knowledge, goals of care can be co-created with patients. Nurses can facilitate patients in the implementation of effective and appropriate coping strategies (Shaha et al., 2011a).

When nursing care is provided within the scope of the theory *The Omnipresence of Cancer* and an understanding of the concept Transitoriness, which weighs heavily

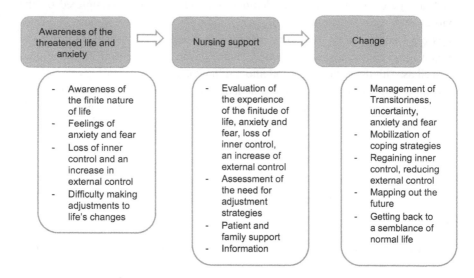

Figure 6.1 Nursing care in Transitoriness

Legend: The first column represents the experience of the finitude of life as articulated in the concept of the Transitoriness. The second column describes the nurses' support. The third column elucidates the expected results following the conceptualization of Transitoriness by patients with nursing support (adapted from Shaha (Shaha, 2016a)).

on patients' minds, patients have an opportunity to talk about their experience of cancer so that feelings of Transitoriness do not become overwhelming (Dolina et al., 2013; Shaha et al., 2006). To do this, it is necessary to provide a favorable time to talk about fears and anxiety. Such support can take place, for example, through interviews using the instrument of Transitoriness. Caregivers must be truly present and attentive to the nonverbal signals patients' present (Shaha et al., 2006; Shaha et al., 2010). The nurse's role manifests itself through information and education given to patients concerning the management of their needs. For example, nurses inform patients about different possibilities associated with treatment modalities and support the patients' selection of choices. Nurses may also include family members, friends and other healthcare professionals in the provision of psychosocial support and care (Shaha et al., 2006; Shaha and Bauer-Wu, 2009).

In summary, the instrument of Transitoriness is grounded in the concept of Transitoriness (Shaha et al., 2006), which in turn is part of the theory *The Omnipresence of Cancer* (Shaha, 2003; Shaha and Cox, 2003). The instrument includes the dimensions of: consciousness, anxiety and change. The instrument of Transitoriness assesses confrontation with and conceptualization of the finitude of life due to a cancer diagnosis and its prognosis. The instrument contains 46 items that are rated using a five-point Likert scale.

Nurses are in a front line position to support the psychosocial needs of cancer patients (Dolina et al., 2013). A cancer disease trajectory includes episodes of acute and chronic manifestations and can be punctuated with grief as well as small victories. Therefore, cancer patients are frequently confronted with the experience of Transitoriness which requires specialized nursing support through adoption of recommendations in the theory, *The Omnipresence of Cancer*.

Case example for practice

The development of the instrument of Transitoriness follows the steps described by DeVellis (2012), thus, ensuring the reliability of content. In future studies steps six and seven will be reconsidered. Subsequently, psychometric validity will be substantiated, allowing for the deployment of the instrument in practice. The development of the instrument of Transitoriness constitutes an important step in the advancement of the theory of *The Omnipresence of Cancer*. With the instrument of Transitoriness it is possible to document cancer patients' experiences of their disease, prognosis and treatment.

Caring for patients throughout their disease trajectory influences nurses and other healthcare professionals in the care they provide. Emotional burden, anxiety and depression can result from caring for cancer patients (de Oliveira et al., 2013). Healthcare professionals may feel a sense of frustration. There is a lack of knowledge about the impact of the existential experience of the finiteness of life and death. Patients' deaths are generally associated with negative feelings, which raise questions about the vulnerability and the fragility of life (Junior et al., 2011). As a result, healthcare professionals face a sense of the finiteness of life experienced by the patients whom they support. In addition, healthcare professionals are personally confronted with questions about their own life's finitude. Education as well as comprehending the theory *The Omnipresence of Cancer*, and, more specifically, the concept of Transitoriness, can address this issue.

Healthcare professionals are encouraged to draw on the theory *The Omnipresence of Cancer* in their practice and to employ the instrument of Transitoriness to identify the experience of the finitude of life cancer patients experience. It is then possible to develop and implement supportive interventions so that patients can manage existential issues in the trajectory of their disease. Cancer patients have psychosocial needs that require attention. Support for day-to-day activities is necessary as well as the provision of comprehensive information about the patients' health condition and the respective medical and nursing care required (Chen et al., 2010). The description and usefulness of the instrument of Transitoriness make it easily transferable in practice. Through findings obtained by the instrument, elements of the theory of *The Omnipresence of Cancer* can be implemented in care settings.

Conclusion

The development of the instrument of Transitoriness meets current expectations of determining support for the psychosocial needs of patients diagnosed with cancer. The instrument offers healthcare professionals a working tool and demonstrates the ability of furthering knowledge of Transitoriness as theoretical concept within the theory *The Omnipresence of Cancer*. The instrument of Transitoriness when utilized in research, education and practice, helps facilitate an understanding of cancer patients' experiences as well as an evaluation of the finitude of life. Research associated with construction of the theory *The Omnipresence of Cancer* and its concept of Transitoriness highlights the need to educate healthcare professionals about the finitude of life and its related experience.

By following the recommendations by DeVellis (2012), the quality of an instrument can be ensured. Adaptations of the methodology have not diminished the quality of the instrument of Transitoriness's development. On the contrary, adaptations have produced significant gains on a methodological level and its content. Further exploration and development of adequate interventions to support patients' experience of Transitoriness have yet to be conducted. To date, validation of the instrument of Transitoriness has been undertaken in Switzerland. There is a need now to extend its validation throughout Europe and elsewhere globally.

References

Adelbratt, S. and Strang, P. 2000. Death anxiety in brain tumour patients and their spouses. *Palliative Medicine*, 14, 499–507.

Barroilhet Diez, S., Forjaz, M. J. and Garrido Landivar, E. 2005. Concepts, theories and psychosocial factors in cancer adaptation. *Actas Espanolas De Psiquiatria*, 33, 390–7.

Blinderman, C. D. and Cherny, N. I. 2005. Existential issues do not necessarily result in existential suffering: lessons from cancer patients in Israel. *Palliative Medicine*, 19, 371–80.

Borges, A. D. V. S., Silva , E. F. D., Mazer, S. M., Toniollo , P. B., Do Valle, E. R. M. and Santos, M. A. D. 2006. Perception of death by oncological patient along its development. *Psicologia em Estudo*, 11, 361–69.

Bouché, O. and Bernhard, U. 2011. *Les annonces en cancérologie: le médecin face au malade: témoignages et repères méthodologiques*. Paris: Springer.

Chen, S. C., Yu, W. P., Chu, T. L., Hung, H. C., Tsai, M. C. and Liao, C. T. 2010. Prevalence and correlates of supportive care needs in oral cancer patients with and without anxiety during the diagnostic period. *Cancer Nursing*, 33, 280–9.

Cohen, M. Z., Williams, L., Knight, P., Snider, J., Hanzik, K. and Fisch, M. J. 2004. Symptom masquerade: understanding the meaning of symptoms. *Supportive Care in Cancer*, 12, 184–90.

Cox, C. R., Reid-Arndt, S. A., Arndt, J. and Moser, R. P. 2012. Considering the unspoken: the role of death cognition in quality of life among women with and without breast cancer. *Journal of Psychosocial Oncology*, 30, 128–39.

De Oliveira, P. P., Amaral, J. G., Viegas, S. M. and Rodrigues, A. B. 2013. The perception of death and dying of professionals working in a long-term care institution for the elderly. *Ciência & Saúde Coletiva*, 18, 2635–44.

Devellis, R. F. 2012. *Scale Development: Theory and Applications*. Thousand Oaks, CA: SAGE.

Dolina, J. V., Bellato, R. and De Araujo, L. F. 2013. Falling ill and dying of a young woman with breast cancer. *Ciência & Saúde Coletiva*, 18, 2671–80.

Dunn, J., Lynch, B., Rinaldis, M., Pakenham, K., McPherson, L., Owen, N., Leggett, B., Newman, B. and Aitken, J. 2006. Dimensions of quality of life and psychosocial variables most salient to colorectal cancer patients. *Psycho-Oncology*, 15, 20–30.

Esbensen, B. A., Swane, C. E., Hallberg, I. R. and Thome, B. 2008. Being given a cancer diagnosis in old age: a phenomenological study. *International Journal of Nursing Studies*, 45, 393–405.

Fortin, F. and Gagnon, J. 2010. *Fondements et étapes du processus de recherche: méthodes quantitatives et qualitatives*. Montréal: Chenelière éducation.

Howard-Anderson, J., Ganz, P. A., Bower, J. E. and Stanton, A. L. 2012. Quality of life, fertility concerns, and behavioral health outcomes in younger breast cancer survivors: a systematic review. *Journal of the National Cancer Institute*, 104, 386–405.

Junior, F. J., Santos, L. C., Moura, P. V., Melo, B. M. and Monteiro, C. F. 2011. Death and dying process: evidences from the literature of nursing. *Revista Brasileira De Enfermagem*, 64, 1122–6.

Lehto, R. H. and Stein, K. F. 2009. Death anxiety: an analysis of an evolving concept. *Research and Theory for Nursing Practice*, 23, 23–41.

Little, M. and Sayers, E. J. 2004a. The skull beneath the skin: cancer survival and awareness of death. *Psycho-Oncology*, 13, 190–8.

Little, M. and Sayers, E. J. 2004b. While there's life . . . hope and the experience of cancer. *Social Science & Medicine*, 59, 1329–37.

McDowell, I. 2006. *Measuring Health: A Guide to Rating Scales and Questionnaires*. New York; Oxford: Oxford University Press.

Morse, J. M., Hupcey, J. E., Mitcham, C. and Lenz, E. R. 1996. Concept analysis in nursing research: a critical appraisal. *Scholarly Inquiry for Nursing Practice*, 10, 253–77.

Pantic, M. 2015. *Déterminer les expériences de la nature transitoire de la vie auprès des personnes multimorbides*. Master of Science in Nursing, University of Lausanne,.

Polit, D. F. and Beck, C. T. 2010. *Essentials of Nursing Research: Appraising Evidence for Nursing Practice*. Philadelphia, PA: Lippincott Williams & Wilkins.

Polit, D. F., Beck, C. T. and Owen, S. V. 2007. Is the CVI an acceptable indicator of content validity? Appraisal and recommendations. *Research in Nursing & Health*, 30, 459–67.

Rust, J. A. and Golombok, S. A. 2015. *Modern Psychometrics: Science of Psychological Assessment (International Library of Psychology)*. London: Routledge.

Shaha, M. 2003. Life with intestinal cancer. A phenomenologic-empirical study. *Pflege*, 16, 323–30.

Shaha, M. 2014. The omnipresence of cancer. In From The Chair of Family Orientated and Community Nursing, F. O. H., Department of Nursing Science (ed.), *Cumulative Thesis in Partial Fulfilment of Obtaining the Venia Legendi for the Subject of Nursing Science of the Faculty of Health, Department of Nursing Science of the University Witten/Herdecke*. Witten/Herdecke, Germany: University of Witten/Herdecke.

Shaha, M. 2016a. The development of a middle-range theory based on phenomenologic research. *QuPuG*, 15, 15–23.

Shaha, M. 2016b. Die Entwicklung einer MR-Theorie basierend auf phänomenologischer Forschung. *QuPuG*, 3, 15–23.

Shaha, M. and Bauer-Wu, S. 2009. Early adulthood uprooted: transitoriness in young women with breast cancer. *Cancer Nursing*, 32, 246–55.

Shaha, M. and Cox, C. L. 2003. The omnipresence of cancer. *European Journal of Oncology Nursing*, 7, 191–6.

Shaha, M., Cox, C. L., Belcher, A. E. and Cohen, M. Z. 2011a. Transitoriness: patients' perception of life after a diagnosis of cancer. *Cancer Nursing Practice*, 10, 24–7.

Shaha, M., Cox, C. L., Cohen, M. Z., Belcher, A. E. and Kappeli, S. 2011b. The contribution of concept development to nursing knowledge? The example of transitoriness. *Pflege*, 24, 361–72.

Shaha, M., Cox, C. L., Hall, A., Porrett, T. and Brown, J. 2006. The omnipresence of cancer: its implications for colorectal cancer. *Cancer Nursing Practice*, 5, 35–9.

Shaha, M., Pandian, V., Choti, M. A., Stotsky, E., Herman, J. M., Khan, Y., Libonati, C., Pawlik, T. M., Schulick, R. D. and Belcher, A. E. 2010. Transitoriness in cancer patients: a cross-sectional survey of lung and gastrointestinal cancer patients. *Supportive Care in Cancer*, 19, 271–9.

Sjovall, K., Gunnars, B., Olsson, H. and Thome, B. 2011. Experiences of living with advanced colorectal cancer from two perspectives – inside and outside. *European Journal of Oncology Nursing*, 15, 390–7.

Streiner, D. L. A., Norman, G. R. A. and Cairney, J. A. 2008. *Health Measurement Scales: A Practical Guide to their Development and Use*. Oxford: Oxford University Press.

Surbone, A., Baider, L., Weitzman, T. S., Brames, M. J., Rittenberg, C. N., Johnson, J. and Group, M. P. S. 2010. Psychosocial care for patients and their families is integral to supportive care in cancer: MASCC position statement. *Support Care Cancer*, 18, 255–63.

Tang, P. L., Chiou, C. P., Lin, H. S., Wang, C. and Liand, S. L. 2011. Correlates of death anxiety among Taiwanese cancer patients. *Cancer Nursing*, 34, 286–92.

Tavares, G. S. 2015. *Développement d'un instrument pour identifier l'expérience de Transitoriness*. Master of Science in Nursing, University of Lausanne,.

Waltz, C. F., Strickland, O. and Lenz, E. R. 2010. *Measurement in Nursing and Health Research*. New York: Springer Pub.

Wild, D., Grove, A., Martin, M., Eremenco, S., Mcelroy, S., Verjee-Lorenz, A., Erikson, P., Translation, I. T. F. F. and Cultural, A. 2005. Principles of Good Practice for the Translation and Cultural Adaptation Process for Patient-Reported Outcomes (PRO) measures: report of the ISPOR task force for translation and cultural adaptation. *Value Health*, 8, 94–104.

Winterling, J., Wasteson, E., Glimelius, B., Sjoden, P. O. and Nordin, K. 2004. Substantial changes in life: perceptions in patients with newly diagnosed advanced cancer and their spouses. *Cancer Nursing*, 27, 381–8.

Woodgate, R. L., West, C. H. and Tailor, K. 2014. Existential anxiety and growth: an exploration of computerized drawings and perspectives of children and adolescents with cancer. *Cancer Nursing*, 37, 146–59.

7 Coping strategies in cancer patients

G. DaRocha and S. Gaillard Desmedt

Introduction

Cancer remains the second cause of medical treatment after cardio-vascular illnesses in Switzerland (Kramis et al., 2013). The risk of developing cancer is increasing in conjunction with an aging population. The incidence of illness in Switzerland is relatively comparable to other European countries (15th out of 40), while the mortality rate is slightly less than the European average. Overall, the prevalence and effect of the cancer will continue to intensify over time. Thanks to scientific advances in diagnostics and therapy, cancer has shifted away from being an acute mortal illness toward a chronic illness. Patients with cancer find themselves in situations of long-term care, with or without clinical symptoms. As cancer has become a chronic illness, there has followed an increase in nursing care to support patients through this long-term process (Kramis et al., 2013).

Cancer, a human experience of vulnerability

Confronting a cancer diagnosis and living with the illness is a challenging experience that affects a significant number of individuals each year (Kramis et al., 2013). To acknowledge one's cancer brings the patient to a state of vulnerability. The announcement of such diagnosis generates an existential crisis with a feeling of life's finiteness (Da Rocha Rodrigues et al., 2014). The person is confronted with thoughts and concerns about death (Adelbratt and Strang, 2000). Psychosocial reactions emerge with the receipt of 'bad news'. A sense of 'Transitoriness' surfaces in the person's thoughts. Transitoriness refers to the feeling of impending finitude of life experienced by patients with cancer. They become aware of the ephemeral nature of existence, understanding that death could occur soon (Winterling et al., 2004). The person can become consumed with feelings of anxiety, fear, distress and anger (Esbensen et al., 2008). It is not unusual for patients, at the prospect of approaching death, to experience an existential crisis (Lehto et al., 2012). The sense of loss, fear, anxiety, panic, despair, loneliness and helplessness can overwhelm people to whom the 'bad news' of cancer is given (Yang et al., 2010; Coyle, 2006). The trajectory of cancer is marked by important stages, each having a significant impact on the patient's well-being and quality of life. The patients, their entourage, including all caregivers, frequently vacillate between uncertainty and hope (Shaha, 2014). Patients' relationships to themselves, to others, to time and to issues of spirituality and religion can change. The cancer experience brings patients toward reflecting on their lives, toward redefining their beliefs and connections in terms of self-identity (Shaha and Cox, 2003). The question of the meaning of life is central to their experience (Stiefel et al., 2008). The beginning of the remission phase is also considered a sensitive moment. Feeling a loss of control that originates from the treatment plan, patients can feel abandoned, lost and fear a relapse (Razavi et al., 2008). To deal with this experience, patients develop and use coping strategies, some of them already well known to patients before the disease, to manage their situation and to adjust to the difficulties imposed by recognising life's finiteness. This adjustment is important to maintain or obtain a better quality of life.

In the theory *The Omnipresence of Cancer* (refer to Chapter 4), the human experience of living with cancer is described. The dimensions of this experience are illuminated in Figure 7.1. With this theory, the psychosocial reactions of

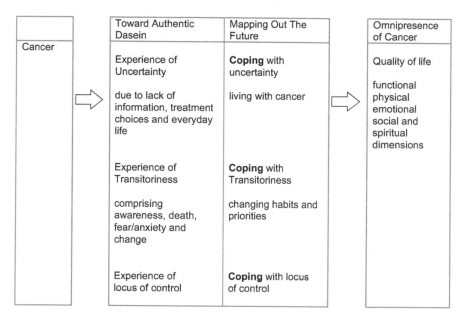

Figure 7.1 The Omnipresence of Cancer (Shaha, 2014; Shaha, 2016)

Legend: A schematic representation of *The Omnipresence of Cancer*. This theory was used as a frame of reference for the studies that will be presented below.

people with cancer and their families, as well as the way they live this situation, are explicated (Shaha, 2014). After having experienced the first phase of being confronted with the cancer diagnosis, a person develops and implements coping strategies in order to carry on toward the future. These endeavours are reflected in the dimensions of a person's quality of life; namely the physical, psychological, social, cultural and spiritual dimensions. In this chapter, the coping strategies that patients use to retain or regain their quality of life and integrate the cancer into all aspects of their daily life will be presented.

Background

Coping

In 1978, Lazarus and Launier delineated the concept of coping. Bruchon-Schweitzer and Dantzer (2003: 2) indicated that based on Lazarus and Launier's delineation, coping strategies are "all the processes that an individual interposes between himself and the event perceived as a threat in order to master, tolerate or diminish its impact on the individual's physical and psychological well-being". These reactions may be cognitive, emotional and/or behavioural; they are meant to maintain the highest level of functioning possible (Razavi et al., 2008). Coping has two primary functions: to make it possible to modify the stress-inducing problem and/or regulate the emotional responses to it. Various coping strategies are used to confront an illness, some are qualified as active – such as problem solving, managing one's emotions, a quest for meaning – others are passive – such as denial, social isolation, avoidance or substance abuse (Bruchon-Schweitzer and Dantzer, 2003).

Faced with the misfortune of the disease, patients re-evaluate and conceptualise new values (Adelbratt and Strang, 2000). Patients decide to embrace life and enjoy it in a new way. It is important to develop coping strategies. Coping strategies such as spirituality and faith help patients reach a sense of inner peace (Jim et al., 2006). A patient who is able to cope with the illness and troubles that accompany cancer and its treatment will perceive the situation differently than those who do not. Those patients that have developed effective coping strategies are able to engage in activities that still have meaning for them (Barroilhet Diez et al., 2005). If patients do not utilise adequate coping strategies, research reflects they experience a loss of meaning and confusion in their lives (Jim et al., 2006).

Numerous research studies have addressed coping styles. Styles studied include optimism, palliative, confrontive, supportive, fatalistic, evasive and emotive. Research studies have illustrated the importance of having optimism when facing cancer. Optimism as a coping style has been shown to be effective in elevating mood in women with breast cancer in China (Zhang et al., 2010), patients with brain cancer in Italy (Palese et al., 2012) and in patients with various forms of cancer in the United States of America (USA) (Felder, 2004). Central to emotions, two styles largely used by cancer patients are the palliative and fatalistic coping styles. Evasive, fatalistic and emotive coping styles have been seen to be the least effective in confronting cancer (Palese et al., 2012; Zhang et al., 2010). Implementation of confrontive and supportive styles are generally favoured (Palese et al., 2012; Felder, 2004; Zhang et al., 2010). Managing one's emotions induced by the cancer experience is listed as a priority compared to styles targeting problem solving. Overall, optimistic and palliative coping styles are widely used and perceived as effective. However, in Italian studies, patients deem optimistic and supportive coping styles to be most effective, not palliative and emotive styles (Palese et al., 2012).

According to Paulham and Bourgeois, individual characteristics, history and perceptions influence choice or capacity to utilise one or more coping styles (Paulham and Bourgeois, 2008). Optimistic (rs = 0.456, p < 0.01), and palliative styles (rs = 0.324, p < 0.01) influence quality of life positively (Guoping and Shan, 2005). A positive relationship has been shown between confrontive and emotive coping styles. These styles are associated with greater self-esteem, satisfaction, vitality and better social functioning with less anxiety and depression in men with prostate cancer (Roesch et al., 2005). Negative relationships have been documented between quality of life and emotive styles, fatalistic styles and, in a lesser way, with evasive styles (Guoping and Shan, 2005).

In a study associated with brain cancer, no correlation was found between age and coping styles of patients (Palese et al., 2012). Furthermore, no correlation was found in relationships between gender and coping in a study conducted in Israel amongst colorectal cancer patients (Goldzweig et al., 2009). Men, particularly if they were not married, utilised strategies associated with a fatalistic style (F = 5.93, p = 0.0154) and powerlessness style (F = 19.83, p = 0.0001) compared to women. Travado et al. (2010) reported higher scores in spirituality amongst patients for combating fatalistic and evasive coping styles.

Coping influences a patient's overall state and functional capacity (Gaillard Desmedt, 2013; Goldzweig et al., 2009). In women with breast cancer (n = 267), (Danhauer et al., 2009) research demonstrated a significant decrease (p < 0.0001) over time in the importance of spirituality, wishful thinking and seeking social support, whereas detachment increased significantly over time (p < 0.0001). Keeping one's feelings to oneself remained a weak coping strategy, whereas cognitive restructuring was highly used by women.

Impaired affective regulation and limited expression of negative feelings were documented in a longitudinal study with newly diagnosed cancer patients (n = 92) (Yu-Chien et al., 2014). No demographic variables were found as explicative factors of coping in a longitudinal predictive study of sarcoma patients (n = 36) (Paredes et al., 2012). More active coping, more social support and religious coping were predictive of a higher meaning in life ($r^2 = 0.17$, $p < 0.01$) in women with breast cancer (n = 167). In addition, these women demonstrated less denial and avoidance (Jim et al., 2006). Poor adjustment was significantly associated with cognitive avoidance and minimal use of approach-based coping responses. Women with passive acceptance and resignation are at risk for poor long-term psychological adjustment (Hack and Degner, 2004).

Coping in surgical and ambulatory chemotherapy treatment departments

DaRocha and Galliard Desmedt undertook three descriptive studies that were conducted, with approval from the respective ethics committees, in two departments of oncology at two university hospitals in the French-speaking part of Switzerland.[1] Table 7.1 reflects an overview of the three studies.

Table 7.1 Overview of the three studies

Design	*Descriptive correlational studies with non-probability purposive sampling*
Sampling	*Inclusion criteria*: patients aged 18 years and over with a cancer diagnosis; fluent in French; in a general state (physical and mental) deemed satisfactory by medical staff; informed consent. *Exclusion criteria*: relapse or in remission.
Data collection	French version of the Jalowiec Coping Scale (Jalowiec, 2003) Measures the degree of use and effectiveness of 60 coping strategies Four-point Likert scale (never used to often used) Organised into eight subscales, i.e., coping styles: confrontive or evasive; optimistic or fatalistic; emotive or palliative; supportant or self-reliant, Cronbach's alpha: 0.88 for the use sub-scale.
Data analysis	'STATA IC' software, Version 12, Normal distribution and homogeneity of variance: Student's t-test or ANOVA test depending on the number of categories, Non-parametric data: Wilcoxon-Mann-Whitney test or Kruskal-Wallis test depending on the number of categories, Pearson's correlation or Spearman's non-parametric test, depending on the variance.

Legend: This table was derived from research undertaken by G. DaRocha and S. Gaillard Desmedt, Master's Degree Students.[1]

Discussion

Findings

In DaRocha's and Galliard Desmedt's research, 88 participants were recruited in hospital outpatient oncology and impatient oncology (n = 48 patients had been visiting an out-patient ambulatory oncology department = group 1; and n = 40 patients had been hospitalised in a surgical ward = group 2). The majority of participants were between 56 and 74 years of age. Men were 53% of the participants; 54% of the participants were retired, and 58% were living as couples. A large number of the participants (39%) had a secondary level education, i.e., apprenticeship. More than half of the participants (n = 54) had digestive cancer. There were a few participants (n = 8) with breast cancer, n = 6 participants had lung cancer and n = 4 participants were diagnosed with gynaecological cancer. A large group (n = 16) of participants presented with other types of cancer. These were haematological, ORL, testicle, brain cancer, melanoma and sarcoma. The majority of the patients (n = 50) were undergoing chemotherapy. Only (n = 4) a few participants were undergoing combination therapy. Table 7.2 demonstrates the sociodemographic characteristics of the participants.

Table 7.2 Participants' sociodemographic characteristics

		All (N = 88)		Group 1 (n = 48)		Group 2 (n = 40)	
		N	%	n	%	n	%
Gender	Women	41	47	22	46	19	47.50
	Men	47	53	26	54	21	52.50
Age	18–36 years	6	7	5	10.50	1	2.50
	37–55 years	18	20	14	29	4	10
	56–74 years	46	52	25	52	21	52.50
	75 and over	18	20	4	8,50	14	35
Marital state	Couple	51	58	33	68.75	18	45
	Single	37	42	15	31.25	22	55
Work	Retired	47	54	19	40	28	70
	Working	36	41	25	52	12	28
	Not working	2	2	1	2	0	0
	Unemployed	1	1	1	2	0	0
	Studying	2	2	2	4	0	0
Level of education	Primary	22	25	6	12.50	16	40
	Secondary	34	39	22	46	12	30
	Tertiary	9	10	5	10.50	4	10
	University	23	26	15	31	8	20

Legend: This table was derived from research undertaken by G. DaRocha and S. Gaillard Desmedt, Master's Degree Students[1].

Table 7.3 JCS use scores (N = 88)

Coping styles	M	SD	Med	Min-Max
Total score (score 0–180)	91.71	17.44	94	43–126
Optimistic (score 0–27)	19.83	4.61	21	3–26
Evasive (score 0–39)	17.84	5.71	18	4–30
Confrontive (score 0–30)	17.34	7.10	18	3–30
Self-reliant (score 0–21)	11.92	4.22	12.50	1–19
Palliative (score 0–21)	8.62	3.01	8.50	0–16
Supportant (score 0–15)	7.79	3.22	8	0–14
Fatalistic (score 0–12)	4.42	2.59	4	0–11
Emotive (score 0–15)	3.94	2.61	4	0–13

Legend: M for mean, SD for standard deviation, MED for median.

Table 7.4 JCS mean item score for use (N = 88)

Rank	Coping style	All (N = 88)		Group 1 (n = 48)	Group 2 (n = 40)
		M (0–3)	SD	M (0–3)	M (0–3)
1	Optimistic	2.20	0.51	2.58	2.10
2	Confrontive	1.73	0.71	2.30	1.80
3	Self-reliant	1.70	0.60	2.23	2.00
4	Supportant	1.56	0.64	2.26	1.50
5	Evasive	1.37	0.44	2.23	1.50
6	Palliative	1.23	0.43	2.36	1.20
7	Fatalistic	1.11	0.65	2.32	1.20
8	Emotive	0.79	0.59	1.85	0.90

Legend: M for mean, SD for standard deviation.

Table 7.5 Most frequently used coping strategies (N = 88)

Rank	Coping strategies	Coping styles	n
1	Try to think positively	Optimistic	71
2	Try to keep your life as normal as possible and not let problem interfere	Optimistic	69
3	Try to keep busy	Palliative	66
3	Think about the good things in your life	Optimistic	66
5	Try to distract yourself by doing something that you enjoy	Palliative	62
5	Try to handle things one step at the time	Confrontive	62
7	Hope that things would get better	Optimistic	61
8	Wish that the problem will go away	Evasive	59
9	Try to keep a sense of humour	Optimistic	56

Legend. Table 7.5 presents the coping strategies that were never used by the participants. For example, 79 of the 88 participants said that they have never used the coping strategy "*Told yourself that the problem was someone else's fault*".

Table 7.6 Never used coping strategies (N = 88)

Rank	Coping strategies	Coping styles	n
1	Told yourself that the problem was someone else's fault	Evasive	79
2	Did something impulsive or risky that you would not usually do	Emotive	73
3	Took a drink to make yourself feel better	Palliative	68
4	Ate or smoked more than usual	Palliative	67
5	Blamed yourself for getting into such a situation	Emotive	65
6	Took out your tensions on someone else	Emotive	64
7	Resigned yourself to the situation because things looked hopeless	Fatalistic	64
8	Took medications to reduce tension	Palliative	63
9	Expected the worst that could happen	Fatalistic	57
10	Put off facing up to the problem	Emotive	56

Legend: This table was derived from research undertaken by G. DaRocha and S. Gaillard Desmedt, Master's Degree Students[1].

Table 7.7 Differences in coping styles used between groups 1 (n = 48) and 2 (n = 40)

Coping styles	Group 1 (n = 48)				Group 2 (n = 40)				Student's t-Test[a]
	M	SD	Min-Max	MED	M	SD	Min-Max	MED	
Total score	89,69	18,41	43–125	96,50	94,20	16,07	50–126	93,50	0,2247
Confrontive	16,79	7,18	3–29	18	18	7,03	3–30	18	0,4299
Evasive	16,85	5,64	4–30	17	19	5,63	7–30	19	0,0756
Optimistic	20,58	3,40	8–26	21	18,92	5,66	3–26	21	0,0934
Fatalistic	4,02	2,16	0–9	3,50	4.90	2,99	0–11	4	0,1139
Emotive	3,52	2,28	0–9	3	4,45	2,91	1–13	4	0,0966
Palliative	9,06	2,87	3–16	8,50	8,10	3,14	0–14	8,50	0,1367
Supportant	8,33	3,22	0–14	9	7,15	3,13	0–12	8	0,0861
Self-reliant	10,48	4,40	1–18	11	13,65	3,27	6–19	13	**<0,0003***

Legend: M for mean, SD for standard deviation, min-max for minimum and maximum, med for median, [a] $^*p < 0,05$.

Coping strategies

The participants in the studies predominantly completed the use-part of the Jalowiec Coping Scale (JCS).

To determine the mean item use score for each coping style, as recommended by Jalowiec (2003), G. DaRocha and S. Gaillard Desmedt divided the subject's raw use score for a specific coping style by the number of coping methods actually used by the subject. The results are presented in Table 7.4. An optimistic coping style is the most frequently used, and an emotive coping style is the least frequently used.

Among the different coping styles, participants used various coping strategies to face up to their illness situation.

The average Cronbach's alpha for the sample of N = 88 was calculated at 0.80 for the use subscale of the JCS. Therefore, the JCS presented a moderate internal consistency in this sample.

The overall coping score differs significantly according to age, marital status, and the level of education of the participants. Hence, the overall coping score is higher in participants aged 75 years and over ($p < 0.0003$), in participants living as a couple or who are married ($p < 0.0246$) and in participants with a high level of education, i.e., with a university degree ($p < 0.0360$). In addition, there are significant differences between the use of the coping styles of participants from group 1 (who were out-patients at an ambulatory oncological department) and participants from group 2 (who had been hospitalised in a surgical oncology department).

Limitations are evident in the study presented above. A descriptive cross-sectional design was selected for this study using a small sample size. Therefore, no cause or effect can be determined. The findings, despite being significant, must be treated with caution. Generalisation is limited. However, the study substantiates the importance of coping in the theory *The Omnipresence of Cancer*. The findings enrich the theory. By exploring coping styles and strategies, it is possible to better understand the patients' experience of living with cancer.

Transitoriness, which constitutes a key concept of the theory, *The Omnipresence of Cancer*, describes a sense of the transitory nature of human life. Persons who are diagnosed with cancer and live with this illness, experience this transitory nature. Questions around death emerge. Transitoriness comprises three attributes, which are: the awareness of the finitude of life, anxiety and change. The first attribute of awareness of the finitude of life consists of three subcategories. These are: threats to life, thoughts of death and leaving the world. The results in the study above demonstrate that threat to life and preoccupation of thought about death are sometimes present from the moment of the diagnosis of cancer. Thoughts about death are part of Toward Authentic Dasein, which constitutes a dimension of the theory *The Omnipresence of Cancer*. Uncertainty and loss of control are also manifested in the studies presented in this chapter.

Findings in these studies point to some facts regarding the more frequently used coping strategies by patients who are diagnosed and live with cancer. Various coping styles are used. Cancer patients primarily use the optimistic coping style. This is similar to older studies using the JCS in cancer patient studies (Felder, 2004; Zhang et al., 2010). Cancer patients also favour confrontive and evasive coping styles (Felder). However, during chemotherapy, cancer patients adopt many other coping styles (Zhang et al., 2010). In G. DaRocha's and S. Gaillard Desmedt's studies, cancer patients also used confrontive and self-reliant coping styles. However, patients undergoing chemotherapy used self-reliant coping styles more often than surgical cancer patients.

Coping strategies used most often are "Try to think positively" and "Try to keep your life as normal as possible and not let the problem interfere". Patients, therefore, wish to keep their hopes up and to have a positive perspective about their illness experience. In G. DaRocha's and S. Gaillard Desmedt's studies, the participants were less inclined to use coping strategies based on expressing their emotions. Findings reinforce the dimension of Mapping Out the Future. It is necessary to support patients in utilising their resources so that they are eventually able to integrate the illness into their daily life. In doing this, it is possible to regain or retain a good quality of life. As part of this quest, patients can find meaning in life, have dynamic and active relationships and mobilise their support systems. In particular, the support systems studied in the research described in this chapter, need further exploration as they have been found to be underdeveloped. Persons diagnosed and living with cancer relinquish control of the situation to others to some extent and also experience uncertainty. Patients live in the moment and have difficulties projecting and making plans for their future. With the help of their chosen coping strategies, patients work toward regaining control of their lives and of returning to a normal daily routine. Hence, the coping strategies adopted form part of the process of finding meaning in the illness situation, which is part of the dimension of Mapping Out the Future. With more understanding of the illness situation, patients can regain control. The experience of Transitoriness influences these actions. Being confronted with the finitude of life comprises living and dying. Transitoriness influences patients and their health, their families and their environment.

Case example for practice

You work in an ambulatory out-patient oncology department, and you are welcoming Mrs La Palma (fictitious name and age), 45 years old, who just finished her last chemotherapy treatment. Mrs La Palma is married and has three young children. She works part time as a teacher at a commercial college. Mrs La Palma was diagnosed six months ago with invasive ductal carcinoma in situ grade III, with T2, N3, M0. She has undergone a mastectomy followed by chemotherapy. After completion of the aforementioned, radiotherapy will start as well as anti-aestrogen hormonal therapy. Mrs La Palma is treated by her gynaecologist and an oncologist.

Underneath her healthy and sunny appearance, Mrs La Palma seems tense and sorrowful. She talks to you about her thoughts about the forthcoming treatment and her preoccupations, the why of this illness and how she could potentially avoid this situation.

While grounding yourself in the theory of *The Omnipresence of Cancer*, you explore with Mrs La Palma her preoccupations and her coping strategies to which she has resorted to confront the forthcoming stage of her illness trajectory and her health experience.

Initially, the health experience and illness situation are explored based on the concepts of the theory. Refer to Table 7.8, which describes the experiences of Uncertainty, Transitoriness and Locus of Control.

Through exploration, you learn that Mrs La Palma has a number of questions concerning her future. The ongoing treatment seems unduly long and arduous. Mrs La Palma wishes to continue to take care of her children and generally return to her normal way of life. She has developed a passion for walking outdoors. This activity helps her to loosen up, to decompress and to regain some energy despite her underlying fatigue. For Mrs La Palma, being a mother makes her happy. She can rely on her husband. His help and support are essential. Mrs La Palma plans to go on a trip with her family after the treatments are over. She also states that imagining her children's future without her is intolerable. Sometimes, she has a feeling that the worst is still to come. It is disappointing when she takes out her anger and her fear on her husband or when she is annoyed with her children.

Through consultation, you have been able to identify several coping strategies for Mrs La Palma. According to the measurement used in the study presented above, the majority of Mrs La Palma 's coping strategies are centred around emotional

Table 7.8 Experiences of Uncertainty, Transitoriness and Locus of Control

Experience of Uncertainty	Stages of the treatment that promote and generate uncertainty: • End of chemotherapy, start of radiotherapy, need for information about the treatments, side effects, therapeutic care plan and efficacy of the chemotherapy. • Impact on daily life, on the organisation of the family, new side effects such as premature menopause or on sexuality, self-esteem, skin alterations etc.
Experience of Transitoriness	• Questions concerning meaning of the illness, of life and of death, of the treatments, becoming aware of the transitory nature of life, the impact of all this on the children, the preoccupations in relation to potential death, a sense of reinforced responsibility, needs in relation to the quality of the relationships with family (her husband, the children) and also support provided by family. • Expression of feelings of anxieties and fears in relation to the future. • New perspectives of the future, personal growth and development, re-evaluated priorities.
Experience of Locus of Control	New feelings of loss of control, readjustment to the therapeutic situation, new projections and ideas for the future.

Legend: This table was derived from research undertaken by G. DaRocha and S. Gaillard Desmedt, Master's Degree Students.[1]

coping. Optimism constitutes a frequently used coping style. For Mrs La Palma, optimism is important, and so she makes use of it. Spirituality also plays an important role for Mrs La Palma, as made evident through her relationship with her family and frequent walks outdoors that help her find meaning in life and lead to a sense of peace. Thoughts of death are present independent of the results of the therapeutic treatments. These thoughts disturb ideas and plans for the future. Mrs La Palma expresses her feelings with crying and anger. As opposed to the participants in the aforementioned study, Mrs La Palma does not seem to find the expression of feelings as a helpful resource. She is afraid that expressing her feelings may lead to being overwhelmed and to increase the worries of her family. Her relationship with her husband is supportive for Mrs La Palma. As opposed to the findings of the above described study, Mrs La Palma does not search actively for others sources of help.

The nursing role in this situation comprises:

- Exploring the lived experience, the feelings of Uncertainty, Transitoriness and Locus of Control.
- Identifying coping strategies used, the resources and the difficulties when confronting this illness situation.
- Supporting coping strategies that are considered effective by Mrs La Palma; validate the invested efforts, widen the perspectives, propose new resources and support.
- Evaluate the results in terms of quality of life, in particular, spiritual well-being.

Conclusion

The theory titled *The Omnipresence of Cancer* offered a solid frame of reference for the studies described in this chapter in order to document the processes and mechanisms that favour the integration of cancer's omnipresence into the life of people concerned. The Case Example for Practice demonstrates the relevance of this theory for use in oncology. This theory guides healthcare professionals into a better understanding of cancer patients' experiences. Subsequently, tailored interventions can be developed and implemented, which help patients develop and use appropriate and purposefully directed coping strategies.

Note

1 The three studies were conducted in partial fulfilment of a Master's of Science in Nursing Degree at the Institute of Higher Education and Research in Healthcare, Faculty of Biology and Medicine, University of Lausanne. Firstly, Maria Goreti Da Rocha (Da Rocha, 2012) conducted a study with patients in a surgical oncology department. This study was followed by the one by Sandra Gaillard Desmedt's research (Gaillard Desmedt, 2013), which was conducted in an outpatient ambulatory oncology department. Thirdly, a descriptive study was conducted compiling the two databases of the previous studies by Leon Cudre (Cudre, 2016). Only data pertaining to coping strategies is presented.

References

Adelbratt, S. and Strang, P. 2000. Death anxiety in brain tumour patients and their spouses. *Palliative Medicine*, 14, 499–507.

Barroilhet Diez, S., Forjaz, M. J. and Garrido Landivar, E. 2005. Conceptos, teorias y factores psicosociales en la adaptaciòn al càncer. *Actas Espanolas De Psiquiatria*, 33, 390–97.

Bruchon-Schweitzer, M. and Dantzer, R. 2003. *Introduction à la psychologie de la santé.* Paris: PUF.

Coyle, N. 2006. The hard work of living in the face of death. *Journal of Pain and Symptom Management*, 32, 266–74.

Cudre, L. 2016. Comparer les stratégies de coping utilisées par les patients traités en première ligne, en ambulatoire et les patients hospitalisés en chirurgie pour un cancer, afain de connaître lesquelles sont déployées les plus fréquemment par les patients pour faire face à la maladie. In IUFRS (ed.), *Masters theses.* Lausanne: University of Lausanne, CHUV Centre Hospitalier Universitaire Vaudois, IUFRS.

Da Rocha Rodrigues, G., Roos, P. and Shaha, M. 2014. Le sentiment de finitude de vie et les stratégies de coping face à l'annonce d'un cancer. *Revue Internationale de soins palliatifs*, 29, 49–53.

Da Rocha, M. G. 2012. Déterminer l'expérience de la proximité de la mort et les stratégies de coping dans des personnes atteintes de cancer. In IUFRS (ed.), *Masters theses.* Lausanne: University of Lausanne, CHUV Centre Hospitalier Universitaire Vaudois, IUFRS.

Danhauer, S. C., Crawford, S. L., Farmer, D. F. and Avis, N. E. 2009. A longitudinal investigation of coping strategies and quality of life among younger women with breast cancer. *Journal of Behavioral Medicine*, 32, 371–9.

Esbensen, B. A., Swane, C. E., Hallberg, I. R. and Thome, B. 2008. Being given a cancer diagnosis in old age: a phenomenological study. *International Journal of Nursing Studies*, 45, 393–405.

Felder, B. E. 2004. Hope and coping in patients with cancer diagnoses. *Cancer Nursing*, 27, 320–4.

Gaillard Desmedt, S. 2013. *Bien-être spirituel et stratégies de coping des patients atteints de cancer en cours de traitement.* Mémoire de master es Sciences en sciences infirmières, Université de Lausanne.

Goldzweig, G., Andritsch, E., Hubert, A., Walach, N., Perry, S., Brenner, B. and Baider, L. 2009. How relevant is marital status and gender variables in coping with colorectal cancer? A sample of middle-aged and older cancer survivors. *Psycho-Oncology*, 18, 866–74.

Guoping, H. and Shan, L. 2005. Quality of life and coping styles in chinese nasopharyngeal cancer patients after hospitalization. *Cancer Nursing*, 28, 179–86.

Hack, T. F. and Degner, L. F. 2004. Coping responses following breast cancer diagnosis predict psychological adjustment three years later. *Psycho-Oncology*, 13, 235–47.

Jalowiec, A. 2003. The Jalowiec coping scale. In O. Strickland and C. Diforio (eds.), *Measurement of Nursing Outcomes. Volume 3: Self Care and Coping.* New York: Springer.

Jim, H. S., Richardson, S. A., Golden-Kreutz, D. M. and Andersen, B. L. 2006. Strategies used in coping with a cancer diagnosis predict meaning in life for survivors. *Journal of Health Psychology*, 25, 753–61.

Kramis, K., Ruckstuhl, B. and Wyler, M. 2013. National strategy against cancer 2014–2017. In Dialog Nationale Gesundheitspolitik (ed.), *Oncosuisse Mandated by Dialog Nationale Gesundheitspolitik.* Bern: Swisscancer.

Lehto, U. S., Ojanen, M., Dyba, T., Aromaa, A. and Kellokumpu-Lehtinen, P. 2012. Impact of life events on survival of patients with localized melanoma. *Psychotherapy and Psychosomatics*, 81, 191–3.

Palese, A., Cecconi, M., Meoreale, R. and Skrap, M. 2012. Pre-oprative stress, anxiety, depression and coping strategies adopted by patients experiencing their first or recurrent brain neoplasm: an explorative study. *Stress and Health*, 28, 416–25.

Paredes, T., Pereira, M., Simões, M. R. and Canavarro, M. C. 2012. A longitudinal study on emotional adjustment of sarcoma patients: the determinant role of demographic, clinical and coping variables. *European Journal of Cancer Care*, 21, 41–51.

Paulham, I. and Bourgeois, M. 2008. *Stress et coping, les stratégies d'ajustement à l'adversité*. Paris, France: PUF.

Razavi, D., Delvaux, N. and Farvacques, C. 2008. Adaptation psychologique: généralités. In D. Razavi and N. Delvaux (eds.), *Précis de psycho-oncologie de l'adulte*. Paris: Masson.

Roesch, S. C., Adams, L., Hines, A., Palmores, A., Vyas, P., Tran, C., Pekin, S. and Vaughn, A. A. 2005. Coping with prostate cancer: a meta-analytic review. *Journal of Behavioral Medecine*, 28, 281–93.

Shaha, M. 2014. The omnipresence of cancer. In From The Chair of Family Orientated and Community Nursing, F. O. H., Department of Nursing Science (ed.), *Cumulative Thesis in Partial Fulfilment of Obtaining the Venia Legendi for the Subject of Nursing Science of the Faculty of Health, Department of Nursing Science of the University Witten/Herdecke*. Witten/Herdecke, Germany: University of Witten/Herdecke.

Shaha, M. 2016. Die Entwicklung einer MR-Theorie basierend auf phänomenologischer Forschung. *QuPuG*, 15, 15–23.

Shaha, M. and Cox, C. L. 2003. The omnipresence of cancer. *European Journal of Oncology Nursing*, 7, 191–6.

Stiefel, F., Krenz, S., Zdrojewski, C., Stagno, D., Fernandez, M., Bauer, J., . . . and Fegg, M. 2008. Meaning in life assessed with the "Schedule for Meaning in Life Evaluation" (SMILE): a comparison between a cancer patient and a student sample. *Support Care Cancer*, 16, 1151–55.

Travado, L., Grassi, L., Gil, F., Martins, C., Ventura, C. and Bairradas, J. 2010. Do spirituality and faith make a difference? Report from the Southern European Psycho-Oncology Study Group. *Palliative and Supportive Care*, 8, 405–13.

Winterling, J., Wasteson, E., Glimelius, B., Sjoden, P. O. and Nordin, K. 2004. Substantial changes in life: perceptions in patients with newly diagnosed advanced cancer and their spouses. *Cancer Nursing*, 27, 381–8.

Yang, W., Staps, T. and Hijmans, E. 2010. Existential crisis and the awareness of dying: the role of meaning and spirituality. *Omega-Journal of Death and Dying*, 61, 53–69.

Yu-Chien, L., Shiow-Ching, S., Wei-Yu, L., Chong-Jen, Y., Pan-Chyr, Y. and Yeur-Hur, L. 2014. Quality of life and related factors in patients with newly diagnosed advanced lung cancer: a longitudinal study. *Oncology Nursing Forum*, 41, E44–55.

Zhang, J., Gao, W., Wang, P. and Wu, Z. H. 2010. Relationships among hope, coping style and social support for breast cancer patients. *Chinese Medical Journal (England)*, 123, 2331–5.

8 Uncertainty in cancer patients

M. Zumstein-Shaha, C. Cox, D. Kelly and K. Talman

Introduction

Cancer remains the second leading cause of death to date, although scientific progress has significantly reduced mortality (WHO, 2017). Lung cancer has become the leading cause of death among all cancer types for both men and women (Torre et al., 2015). In the US, the UK, and Switzerland, cancer remains the second leading cause of death, which is only being surpassed by cardiovascular diseases (American Cancer Society, 2017; Arndt et al., 2016). Having a diagnosis of cancer remains a threat to life, which can lead to negative experiences such as loss or uncertainty as well as positive experiences such as adopting a healthier lifestyle (Litzelman et al., 2017). Uncertainty is defined as "the inability to determine the meaning of illness-related events. It is a cognitive state created when the individual cannot adequately structure or categorize an illness event because of insufficient cues" (Mishel, 2014: 53). Uncertainty related to the disease trajectory and uncertainty related to daily and existential issues have also been identified (Shaha et al., 2008). Uncertainty is recognized as a frequent experience in patients who are diagnosed with cancer (Cahill et al., 2012). In particular, a lack of comprehensible and comprehensive information promotes uncertainty leading to negative disease trajectory experiences (Kazer et al., 2013; Donovan and Glackin, 2012; Cahill et al., 2012; Campbell-Enns and Woodgate, 2016).

In 2008, a concept analysis of uncertainty was explicated by Shaha et al. Since 2008, no new concept analysis of uncertainty has been published. In the theory *The Omnipresence of Cancer*, uncertainty is seen as one of its main concepts. The purpose of this chapter, therefore, is to describe the experience of uncertainty in relation to this theory. As the theory focuses predominantly on patients newly diagnosed and living with cancer, the description of uncertainty will be explicated in relation to this patient group. An evolutionary concept analysis as proposed by Rodgers (1989) is presented. Concept analysis forms the foundation for theory building. In this chapter, due to the structure of the concept analysis process, some aspects of narrative are explicated in a duplicative manner.

Background

Uncertainty constitutes an important reaction in cancer patients. In 2014, Mishel updated her "Theories of uncertainty in illness" (Mishel, 2014). The Mishel Uncertainty in Illness Scale (MUIS) has been employed in a number of studies with cancer patients and has been translated into several languages, including Persian (Hagen et al., 2015; Giammanco et al., 2015; Hall et al., 2014; Lin et al., 2012; Parker et al., 2013; Hoth et al., 2015; Bailey et al., 2011; Kurita et al., 2013; Jeon et al., 2016; Zhang et al., 2015; Sajjadi et al., 2014; Syrjala et al., 2016). At present, uncertainty is generally being measured through the MUIS (Hagen et al., 2015).

The theory "Uncertainty in Illness" by Mishel (2014) is often employed in caring for patients, in particular, to represent or support a nursing perspective of caring (Mishel et al., 2009; Checton et al., 2012; Kazer et al., 2010; Suzuki, 2012). This theory proposes a definition of uncertainty and maintains that persons who are confronted with uncertainty appraise their situation to identify known and unknown aspects of their illness. Drawing on this appraisal, persons determine the quality of uncertainty. It is identified whether the experienced uncertainty is a threat or a potential. Generally, uncertainty is considered neither good nor bad. Subsequently, persons develop or employ mobilizing or buffering coping strategies and affect controlling strategies (Mishel, 2014: 57). Providing comprehensible and comprehensive information about the disease and cancer trajectory constitute important interventions within Mishel's uncertainty in illness theory (Mishel, 2014).

Another theory addressing uncertainty is the "Uncertainty Management Theory" (UMT) by Brashers (2001, 2007) and Brashers et al. (2000) (cited by: Rains and Tukachinsky, 2015a: 339). Similar to Mishel's Uncertainty in Illness theory, the UMT maintains that uncertainty occurs "when details of situations are ambiguous, complex, unpredictable or probabilistic; when information is unavailable or inconsistent; and when people feel insecure in their own state of knowledge or the state of knowledge in general" (Brashers, 2001: 478, cited by: Rains and Tukachinsky, 2015a: 339). As part of the UMT, the person facing uncertainty also evaluates it in view of potential threats or added value. Uncertainty here, is also neutral; neither positive nor negative. Persons attribute values based on their appraisal and of having determined potential threats or benefits. Uncertainty as a threat is negative and leads to increased fear and anxiety. Persons may choose to avoid the situation provoking uncertainty for example. When a person considers uncertainty to be an opportunity, hope is experienced, and a positive outlook is promoted. There is a difference between the current and actual level of uncertainty as experienced in each situation and the amount of uncertainty a person would like to feel. The UMT therefore recommends to assess the level of uncertainty a person experiences, to determine the amount and type of support that are needed. Within the UMT framework, avoiding information or deliberately looking for information are important strategies to deal with uncertainty (Rains and Tukachinsky, 2015a).

In relation to a cancer diagnosis, uncertainty arises from the moment a cancer diagnosis is suspected or impending and lasts throughout the disease trajectory (Campbell-Enns and Woodgate, 2016). There is uncertainty regarding the impact of the disease on one's body image, related to waiting for the treatments to begin, to treatment outcomes or to decision making (Mollica et al., 2016; Pacian et al., 2012; Newcomb et al., 2016; Donovan and Glackin, 2012). In particular, symptoms are viewed as contributing to uncertainty (Cahill et al., 2012). Due to the cancer diagnosis, persons are faced with changing daily demands and needs. Daily life and familiar supportive structures are overturned and need to be reconstructed or adjusted (Zhang et al., 2015; Donovan and Glackin, 2012). The experience of uncertainty can lead to a reduced quality of life, reduced ability to self-care and additionally influence a person's coping with the disease situation (Zhang et al., 2015; Taneja, 2013; Lang et al., 2013; Donovan and Glackin, 2012). Behavioral and psychosocial interventions as well as spirituality are viewed as helpful to counter the experience of uncertainty (Mollica et al., 2016).

Although uncertainty has been described on several occasions, updates are important to improve care (Morse et al., 1996). Uncertainty as a concept in patients who are newly diagnosed with cancer and therefore early on in their disease trajectory or treatment has yet to be fully described. Therefore, an evolutionary concept analysis is presented below related to uncertainty in newly diagnosed cancer patients involved in their initial treatments. For this concept analysis, PubMed and Medline/Embase databases were searched as well as Web of Knowledge. Articles included in the analysis addressed newly diagnosed cancer patients in initial treatment. A few publications spanning from initial treatment to end-of-life were also included. In addition to the aforementioned, the experience of uncertainty required description. Articles treating psychosocial issues were included provided uncertainty was mentioned. The retained publications were all in English. All publications associated with treating quality of life or uncertainty in relation to measuring or diagnostic procedures or that included the perspective of the relatives or the healthcare professionals were excluded.

Medline/Embase was searched using the terms uncertainty and primary cancer as major headings combined with initial treatment. The search was limited to the publications that had emerged between 2008 and 2017. A total of 74 articles were found that were retained. The following search strings were applied in Medline: uncertainty, neoplasms, and therapeutics as MeSH (Medical Subject Headings) terms. The term therapy was used as a subheading. The following terms were included, namely therapy, treatment, therapeutics, uncertainty, psychosocial, and cancer. These findings were limited to publications between 2008 and 2017. The limitation of 2008 was applied as the comprehensive literature review on uncertainty was published then (Shaha et al., 2008). A total of three articles were found and retained. The same search string was applied to Web of Knowledge, but none of the search yielded new articles that could be retained.

A final search was conducted in PubMed with uncertainty and neoplasms used as MeSH terms, in association with cancer as well as psychosocial. This search was also limited to publications that had emerged between 2008 and 2017. A total of 172 articles were found of which a total of 27 were retained. Overall, 62 articles pertaining to uncertainty in adult cancer patients at the beginning of their disease trajectory and in treatment were found. All these 101 articles were published after 2008. These articles were analyzed using the evolutionary concept analysis approach described by Rodgers (1989).

Discussion

A total of seven scientific specialties were identified. Most the articles were from nursing. Only a few articles were from related fields such as sociology or economics.

The term "uncertainty" is predominantly used in the literature. Surrogate terms are rare. Occasionally, "unexpectedness" is employed (Lim et al., 2015). Uncertainty is viewed as a symptom (Elphee, 2008; Hagen et al., 2015) and/or as an important part of psychological or psychosocial issues (Bailey et al., 2014; Bogaarts et al., 2012). Occasionally, uncertainty is subsumed in fear, anxiety, depression, or distress (Beach and Dozier, 2015; Brown and Oetzel, 2016; Ellis et al., 2013; Horrill, 2016; Syrjala et al., 2016; Sautier et al., 2014).

Antecedents (application)

Uncertainty is associated with any type of cancer, from early adulthood to older age (Black et al., 2015; Sautier et al., 2014; Mazor et al., 2013; Beach and Dozier, 2015; Hammond et al., 2015; Aldaz et al., 2016; Grimsbo et al., 2011). The

Table 8.1 Overview of specialties

Nursing:	26
Oncology, Medicine	14
Communication	4
Psychology	13
Public health	2
Sociology	1
Economics	2
Total	**62**

diagnoses of breast and prostate cancer are frequently studied (Zhang et al., 2015; Jones et al., 2015; Kennedy et al., 2008; Brown and Oetzel, 2016; Schumm et al., 2010; Mollica et al., 2016; Parker et al., 2016; Horrill, 2016). Among the group of breast cancer patients (Campbell-Enns and Woodgate, 2016; Edib et al., 2016), there are specific foci on patients with ductal carcinoma in situ (Kennedy et al., 2010), with neoadjuvant treatment (Kyranou et al., 2014; Hagen et al., 2015), or with triple negative breast cancer (TNBC) subtype (Turkman et al., 2016). This final cancer category is extremely aggressive and includes high recurrence and mortality rates. Young African-American women carrying the BRCA1 gene are more often affected than other women. There are limited treatment options for these patients. These patients identify uncertainty as "insecurity", i.e., "flying without a net" (Turkman et al., 2016).

Prostate cancer patients are represented within the newly diagnosed and patients under active surveillance (Brown and Oetzel, 2016; Schumm et al., 2010; Mollica et al., 2016; Parker et al., 2016; Horrill, 2016) or patients treated surgically with a follow-up on the level of their prostate-specific antigen (PSA) (Bailey et al., 2014). Patients with prostate cancer qualify for active surveillance if their disease is considered low-risk (Horrill, 2016).

Recently, there are also studies involving diagnoses such as head and neck cancer, brain cancer, lung or hematological cancer (Hendriksen et al., 2015; Kurita et al., 2013; Cavers et al., 2013; Syrjala et al., 2016; Ghodraty-Jabloo et al., 2016; Parker et al., 2013; Wong et al., 2013; Haisfield-Wolfe et al., 2012). There are also studies involving gastrointestinal cancer (Al Qadire, 2014; Ellis et al., 2013; Jeon et al., 2016; Beesley et al., 2016). A few studies involve patients with rarer forms of cancer, such as indolent lymphoma (Elphee, 2008), malignant pleural mesothelioma (Arber and Spencer, 2013), and Pseudomyxoma peritonei (PMP) (Witham et al., 2008).

Uncertainty in cancer patients in treatment (use)

Uncertainty exists, besides other manifestations such as shock, anxiety or fear, from the moment of a cancer diagnosis throughout the disease (Kazer et al., 2013; Stenberg et al., 2012; Grimsbo et al., 2011; Lambert et al., 2012). Directly after the confirmation of a cancer diagnosis and early in the trajectory uncertainty is prominent (Arber and Spencer, 2013: Al; Qadire, 2014; Cavers et al., 2013; Mollica et al., 2016; Beach and Dozier, 2015; Brown and Oetzel, 2016; Parker et al., 2013; Kennedy et al., 2008). Uncertainty remains at high level beyond treatments (Haisfield-Wolfe et al., 2012; Lin et al., 2015). Patients with high uncertainty have a reduced performance status (Lin et al., 2013). In relation to a poor prognosis, uncertainty can persist after diagnosis and treatment (Ghodraty-Jabloo et al., 2016; Jeon et al., 2016). Cancer patients with more aggressive or advanced disease have reduced hope. For them, coping is challenging (Cavers et al., 2013). Uncertainty is increased in patients with rare types of cancer or aggressive disease as there are difficult diagnostic processes involved and challenges in finding the most suitable treatment in view of having a restrained possibility for cure (Turkman et al., 2016; Witham et al., 2008). Cancer diagnoses signify several examinations and test, which are often carried out in a variety of medical departments. Patients meet a variety of healthcare professionals and have to navigate a complex healthcare system. In these situations, the level of uncertainty increases (Elphee, 2008; Hammond et al., 2015; Mazor et al., 2013; Kennedy et al., 2008).

Cancer patients and families often experience information deficits. Sufficient information about the disease, its evolution, its impact on life, treatment success, effects, or side effects, as well as life beyond the diagnosis and the treatments are rarely available (Al Qadire, 2014; Schumm et al., 2010; Ellis et al., 2013; Cavers et al., 2013; Brown and Oetzel, 2016; Elphee, 2008; Hendriksen et al., 2015; Kennedy et al., 2008). There is a limited possibility of gauging remaining time in life and thus looking beyond the diagnostic and treatment phase. Each contributes to uncertainty (Hendriksen et al., 2015). Making decisions under such circumstances is challenging (Schumm et al., 2010; Goh et al., 2012; Hanratty et al., 2013). Anti-cancer treatments can have various outcomes, thereby provoking uncertainty. There are no rights or wrongs regarding decisions for or against treatments. Everything around the cancer diagnosis can be confusing (Schumm et al., 2010).

Cancer patients can experience numerous symptoms or side-effects due to the disease and its treatments (Ghodraty-Jabloo et al., 2016; Grimsbo et al., 2011). Vague symptoms that are not evident persistently such as fatigue provoke uncertainty about treatments, disease prognosis and quality of life (Kurita et al., 2013; Bailey et al., 2014; Cahill et al., 2012). The more symptoms are present, the more uncertainty is found (Haisfield-Wolfe et al., 2012). High levels of psychosocial distress, behavioral and psychological manifestations of depression impair patients' tolerance. Ambiguity about the disease is increased (Kurita et al., 2013), leading to uncertainty. Patients undergoing treatment experience high uncertainty regarding the evolution of symptom and symptom severity (Lin et al., 2015). Mood modifies uncertainty, which can reduce perceived symptom severity. The various treatment phases, changing or losing work due to the disease are significant predictors for uncertainty (Lin et al., 2015). Sometimes, patients employ avoidance to cope with uncertainty, which may have a detrimental effect (Kurita et al., 2013).

Before starting treatment there are waiting periods, which elicit high uncertainty and distress (Donovan and Glackin, 2012). The normalit of life is disrupted. Patients ask themselves about outcomes of the treatments or life after completion of the treatment. Here, uncertainty is characteristic of the period from diagnosis beyond completion of the treatment. After treatment, patients ask themselves about recurrence or disease progression (Lang et al., 2013).

A cancer diagnosis and its treatment signify unpredictability, call forth the question of survival and potential death. Patients are confronted with the transitory nature of life (Hendriksen et al., 2015; Aldaz et al., 2016; Ellis et al., 2013) and existential uncertainty (Hammond et al., 2015). Time is viewed as limited (Hendriksen et al., 2015). Uncertainty is associated with the experience of finitude of life (Transitoriness) and locus of control (r=0.3267, p=0.0002/r=0.1994, p=0.0252, respectively) (Shaha et al., 2010). Quality of life is negatively influenced by uncertainty (r=-0.4929, p=0.0000) (Shaha et al., 2010). Fear and uncertainty seem to abate slightly during treatment as patients attach hope (Ellis et al., 2013). Cancer implies expectations of remission or of preventing disease progression and unknown changes leading to worry (Hendriksen et al., 2015). It has been found that hopeful patients mobilizing spiritual resources are better able to cope with uncertainty (Cavers et al., 2013). Spirituality reduces uncertainty and stress (Mollica et al., 2016).

An important part of a cancer diagnosis is regular and systematic monitoring visits after completion of the anti-cancer treatments. Patients identify information and knowledge deficits in relation to these follow-up visits. Often, the monitoring results are not conveyed within a reasonable time frame. There is much time to chew over the situation and to worry. A cancer diagnosis raises questions about the future (Ellis et al., 2013; Beesley et al., 2016; Edib et al., 2016; Watson et al., 2015; Hanratty et al., 2013).

Uncertainty influences recovery from treatments. In conjunction with this, high levels of uncertainty reduce an experienced quality of life in cancer patients and their spouses. Due to the cancer diagnosis, patients and their families face life's finitude. Families' thoughts and feelings vacillate between the imminence of death and the wish for a full recovery. In view of the confrontation with life's finitude, families prepare for a future without the sick family member. The how, the when, and in what way changes occur are unknown. Many new roles and changes are attached to life beyond the treatments when in view of potential death (Hendriksen et al., 2015; Stenberg et al., 2012). Social support and improved dyadic communication reduce uncertainty in cancer patients, their spouses, and families (Song et al., 2011).

Issues regarding the medical treatment plan and the disease situation, including the prognosis and patients' psychosocial responses to the disease, constitute important areas of communication between healthcare professionals and patients. Goals differ between patients and healthcare professionals, which contributes to uncertainty (Brataas et al., 2010). Sometimes, healthcare professionals become distant and removed from patients who may wish to address uncertainty (Beach and Dozier, 2015). Patients can feel excluded from exchanges between healthcare professionals and families. By not considering the patient's perspective, health-care professionals foster the patient's experience of exclusion. Thus, patients may feel like outsiders (Hammond et al., 2015).

Prostate cancer

Uncertainty often arises in conjunction with a treatment option of engaging in "active surveillance". In active surveillance, there is uncertainty regarding information about the disease itself, the potential influence of lifestyle, associated changes and/or repeated examinations such as prostate biopsies. Waiting for the disease to potentially develop is associated with considerable stress for patients, their spouses, and families. These uncertainties can influence treatment adherence in significant ways. Delaying immediate treatment in active surveillance has the advantage of maintaining quality of life, which can lead to an improved perspective related to eventual anti-cancer treatments. Men undergoing active surveillance face issues such as suspecting there will be no treatment effect, that the disease will progress, or that there will be subsequent morbidities due to treatment (Kazer et al., 2013; Horrill, 2016; Parker et al., 2016; Goh et al., 2012; Lambert et al., 2012; Oliffe et al., 2009). It is evident from the literature that uncertainty affects men's quality of life and is also a predictor of psychological distress; notably depression, anxiety, and hostility. Men frequently fear that under active surveillance, disease progression may be discovered too late and that curative treatment may no longer be possible. Research indicates that patients under active surveillance feel left alone; they have many questions and no reference person to provide answers (Horrill, 2016; Parker et al., 2016; Oliffe et al., 2009). The PSA, which is an indicator for prostate cancer, can vary and not necessarily be a clear indicator for the disease; thus, uncertainty is increased (Bailey et al., 2014). Uncertainty associated with active surveillance has also been shown to lead to patients opting for more invasive treatment sooner than recommended (Oliffe et al., 2009).

Breast cancer

Women who have or have had breast cancer experience amongst other issues such as fatigue and low sexual or reproductive interest. This is shown to be related to uncertainty and anxiety regarding potential recurrence (Campbell-Enns and Woodgate, 2016). Women demonstrate moderate to high levels of uncertainty about their future (Campbell-Enns and Woodgate, 2016; Kennedy et al., 2008). Uncertainty is evident from a cancer diagnosis onward. In particular, newly diagnosed patients have difficulties adjusting to the disease situation as they have limited knowledge about the disease or treatment options. Patients with a low level of education and high economic pressure find it challenging to cope with their illness situation (Kyranou et al., 2014; Zhang et al., 2015; Edib et al., 2016; Hanratty et al., 2013; Campbell-Enns and Woodgate, 2016; Kennedy et al., 2008). Self-care behaviour in women with breast cancer influences adaptation to the disease situation. High levels of uncertainty and low levels of self-efficacy have been found to limit self-care behaviour (Zhang et al., 2015). Occasionally, women who have or have had breast cancer do not know the kinds of support they should request during periods of stress that will assist in resolving aspects of their uncertainty (Campbell-Enns and Woodgate, 2016).

Colorectal cancer

Being diagnosed with colorectal cancer is associated with a number of issues that are not expected such as the treatment and its influence on patients' lives. This is particularly true when patients face the potential of having a stoma. Uncertainty becomes evident as soon as the cancer diagnosis is made and treatment options are discussed. Literature has shown that patients need information about a stoma and its associated issues before returning home. Without this patients struggle with uncertainty about how to manage their situation. With good information at hand, patients are better able to manage unforeseeable situations and demonstrate lower levels of uncertainty and anxiety. The same applies to knowledge about medication and lifestyle. Patients need to be prepared before discharge from hospital about lifestyle changes in order to promote adaptation to the demands of the disease situation avoid the development of uncertainty. Research has demonstrated that it is not considered helpful to receive information shortly before discharge, as patients are unable to assimilate the information and experience hightened levels of uncertainty (Lim et al., 2015; Park et al., 2014).

Outcomes of uncertainty and potential interventions (significance)

Uncertainty leads to patients knowing they have to accept the cancer diagnosis and find ways to live with it. Nevertheless, patients wish for their previous (normal) life to resume (Brown and Oetzel, 2016). In the case of aggressive types of cancer, uncertainty regarding outcomes promotes living on a day-to-day basis. Patients worry (Arber and Spencer, 2013). Being diagnosed with advanced cancer often means that patients have limited hope. In this situation, uncertainty influences patients' adherence to and recovery from treatment. Patients experience uncertainty beyond the treatment period as they continue to worry about the return of the disease. Coping with uncertainty presents a challenge (Cavers et al., 2013) and influences patients' ability to adapt to the disease in daily life (Haisfield-Wolfe et al., 2012; Goh et al., 2012).

Uncertainty provokes anxiety, fear, and distress, reduces hope and quality of life (Lang et al., 2013; Elphee, 2008; Suzuki, 2012; Hendriksen et al., 2015;

Parker et al., 2013; Arber and Spencer, 2013; Syrjala et al., 2016; Campbell-Enns and Woodgate, 2016; Oliffe et al., 2009). A cancer diagnosis can lead to "distancing oneself from one's self-concept" (Wong et al., 2013: 1055). For quality of life and fear of progression uncertainty acts as a predictor (Parker et al., 2013) as evidenced in this chapter associated with prostate cancer. High levels of uncertainty in combination with increased anxiety can increase patients' motivation to search for information and to try to find answers (Beach and Dozier, 2015; Goh et al., 2012). Uncertainty influences self-care behavior in patients (Zhang et al., 2015). In some cases, uncertainty can lead to accepting invasive treatment sooner than necessary (Oliffe et al., 2009), as mentioned previously in this chapter.

A cancer diagnosis is associated with life's finitude and calls forth existential concerns (Hammond et al., 2015; Aldaz et al., 2016). Thus, patients begin the process of rearranging their outlook, changing priorities and/or developing new ones. In order to find a way to accept the disease situation, patients often "take things as they come" (Aldaz et al., 2016: 7). Finally, research has indicated patients value discussions with health professionals (Aldaz et al., 2016) in order to increase their knowledge of how to manage their illness and activities of daily living.

Research has shown the future is difficult for patients to envision. The disease and its uncertain trajectory influence everyday living, including planning for the future. Research indicates future roles are difficult to foresee or to prepare for (Hendriksen et al., 2015; Beesley et al., 2016; Edib et al., 2016; Hanratty et al., 2013). Thus, a patient's sense of dignity can be reduced (Sautier et al., 2014).

Interventions to reduce uncertainty

To cope with uncertainty, comprehensible information tailored to the patients' and the families' needs is considered a key intervention (Cavers et al., 2013; Parahoo et al., 2015; Lim et al., 2015; Kazer et al., 2013; Stenberg et al., 2012). Information needs to address the specificities of the disease, the treatment and its effects or side effects and any aspects of daily life that may change because of the disease or its treatment (Turkman et al., 2016; Lim et al., 2015; Horrill, 2016; Kazer et al., 2013). Checking regularly to discern whether patients and their families have grasped the information can contribute to reduced uncertainty (Beach and Dozier, 2015; Stenberg et al., 2012). Information needs to be provided in a structured way, addressing concrete issues, including symptom management (Ellis et al., 2013; Cahill et al., 2012). Information on disease-related issues needs comprehensive preparation on the part of the healthcare professional so that all patient questions and issues can be addressed. It is recommended provision of information is carefully managed over a period of time and not at the last minute (Lim et al., 2015) in order to ensure the patient has assimilated and understands the information provided. Engaging in this activity will reduce levels of uncertainty and promote the development of coping strategies.

It is imperative that uncertainty is systematically and regularly assessed from the diagnosis of cancer onward. It is recommended that the healthcare practitioner assess patients' needs, symptoms, and levels of uncertainty together with anxiety, distress, and dignity as well as coping mechanisms (Beach and Dozier, 2015; Sautier et al., 2014; Syrjala et al., 2016; Ellis et al., 2013; Ghodraty-Jabloo et al., 2016; Jeon et al., 2016; Lin et al., 2015; Shaha et al., 2010; Brataas et al., 2010). These evaluations need to be carried out regularly across the disease trajectory (Beach and Dozier, 2015; Lin et al., 2015; Shaha et al., 2010). Based on these assessments, healthcare professionals will be able to develop and provide adequate support and reassurance. It is important to address the patient's inability to tolerate uncertainty associated with the cancer diagnosis and the patient's adoption of coping strategies that promote avoidance associated with distress and depression (Kurita et al., 2013). Some patients also attempt to refrain from identifying with the stereotype of "cancer patient" by "distancing" themselves from it to cope with the cancer diagnosis (Wong et al., 2013: 1055). Having high uncertainty reinforces these behaviors and reduces the possibility of adopting adequate coping strategies (Wong et al., 2013). The provision of effective psychological interventions and symptom management beyond the treatment period is essential in reducing uncertainty (Ghodraty-Jabloo et al., 2016; Jeon et al., 2016; Song et al., 2011). Some patients are eager to obtain information by themselves. These efforts need to be encouraged by healthcare professionals (Horrill, 2016).

Offering hope and spiritual support are effective in reducing uncertainty (Cavers et al., 2013), as well as helping the patient find meaning during the disease process (Lang et al., 2013). As a result, patients are better able to make decisions concerning the disease and associated treatments (Mollica et al., 2016). In some cases, the inclusion of a spiritual or religious advisor can be helpful (Syrjala et al., 2016). Helping patients to identify their support network and promoting these networks contributes to reduced uncertainty and the development of better coping mechanisms (Brown and Oetzel, 2016; Elphee, 2008; Wong et al., 2013).

It has been identified that patients do not necessarily receive adequate social support from the initial diagnosis onward. Palliative care is frequently not provided at the beginning of a cancer trajectory (Arber and Spencer, 2013). Helping patients identify a social network and social support as well as providing palliative care early in the cancer trajectory are considered important helpful elements in reducing uncertainty, particularly when support can be provided by previous cancer survivors (Arber and Spencer, 2013).

In order to better cope with the existential aspects of a cancer diagnosis, patients try to find a way to accept the disease situation and to "take things as they come" (Aldaz et al., 2016: 7). It can be helpful for patients to talk about this experience with healthcare professionals or write about it (Hammond et al., 2015; Aldaz et al., 2016; Shaha et al., 2010). For some patients, interventions are needed that foster maintaining employment or finding more adequate employment (Suzuki, 2012). Ultimately, a patient's quality of life and sense of well-being can be maintained or even improved when appropriate strategies are impelmented by health-care providers (Aldaz et al., 2016).

As part of the cancer trajectory, patients and their families engage in a unique relationship with healthcare professionals. Depending on the amount and quality of information provided, this relationship can improve or worsen a patient's levels of uncertainty. Comprehensive information targeting patients' needs as well as questions from patients' families is essential in fostering a positive relationship which subsequently reduces uncertainty (Mazor et al., 2013; Kazer el al., 2013). In contrast, less tailored or limited information is not well received and can increase uncertainty patients experience. Good relationships between patients, families, and healthcare professionals promote coping with uncertainty. Interventions targeting the provision of information and a positive supportive relationship with healthcare professionals are important as they can contribute to better care (Mazor et al., 2013). Patients wish for healthcare professionals to acknowledge their feelings, reactions, and experiences (Turkman et al., 2016). Research has shown without exception that support and reassurance from health-care professionals are important factors in the early disease trajectory (Cavers et al., 2013; Beach and Dozier, 2015; Elphee, 2008; Lang et al., 2013). It is recommended that healthcare professionals adapt care priorities by taking into account patients' preferences (Kazer et al., 2013). Engaging in shared goal setting with patients promotes addressing the ability to address patients' uncertainty (Brataas et al., 2010). In relation to healthcare professionals giving support to patients who experience uncertainty, the provision education is necessary (Elphee, 2008; Lang et al., 2013). Nurses are considered well placed to provide support to patients experiencing uncertainty (Kazer et al., 2013). Developing and implementing guidelines based on evidence are important in order to offer adequate interventions to patients (Donovan and Glackin, 2012; Turkman et al., 2016; Lang et al., 2013).

A variety of interventions have been identified for targeting and managing uncertainty, fostering coping, and providing general support to patients (Bailey et al., 2014; Lin et al., 2013; Lin et al., 2012). Among these are nursing support groups or interventions based on mindfulness as well as interventions targeting cognitive refraiming, self-care or self-efficacy (Bailey et al., 2014; Parahoo et al., 2015; Zhang et al., 2015; Carlson, 2016). However, it is important to keep in mind that research has demonstrated that many psychosocial interventions, particularly those targeting patients with prostate cancer evidence limited effectiveness (Parahoo et al., 2015). Further research is important (Kyranou et al., 2014) to determine the best way to support this group of patients (Witham et al., 2008; Horrill, 2016).

Outcomes

Uncertainty is a pervasive experience for patients when a cancer diagnosis is made. A primary indicator of uncertainty is the patient's lack of konwledge about the disease and its evolution. Uncertainty has been defined by researchers as being neutral as well as positive and negative (Rains, 2014; Rains and Tukachinsky, 2015b; Mishel, 2014). Its levels have been identified as moderate to high in cancer patients. There are indications that these levels persist beyond the cancer treatment. However, the levels of uncertainty require further exploration across the disease trajectory. Cancer patients identify three main sources of uncertainty. Firstly, there is uncertainty associated with an information deficit concerning the disease and its evolution. Secondly, patients are uncertain about the treatment and its side-effects as well as its impact on daily life. Finally, cancer has an existential impact as patients are coming face to face with the finitude of their lives.

Uncertainty is associated with patients' symptoms and influences patients' and families' quality of life and well-being. High uncertainty levels can influence the symptom experience, reduce coping as well as recovery from treatment. It is therefore imperative that effective interventions are developed and implemented to reduce uncertainty and to provide ways for patients to adapt and find meaning in the disease situation. Several interventions aiming at reducing uncertainty or managing it are known, as previously indicated in this chapter. However, the full effectiveness of these interventions has yet to be established. Further research into the experience of uncertainty across the disease trajectory is necessary to further explicate its presence and manifestation in the two dimensions Toward Authentic Dasein and Mapping Out the Future proposed by the theory *The Omnipresence of Cancer*.

Case example for practice

A 60-year-old married gentleman with no children presented with a diagnosis of prostate cancer. The gentleman is educated at apprenticeship level and is working at the local bank. He was diagnosed with low risk prostate cancer three months ago. The primary diagnosis of prostate cancer was determined through a PSA level of <4ng/mL (adjusted for volume). The prostate cancer had a tumor focus of <3 mm. Active surveillance was considered the appropriate treatment option for this gentleman. Thus, this gentleman began consultation with a urologist every six months, which included clinical examinations, digital rectal examinations, and measurement of PSA and testosterone levels. In addition, all current medications were reviewed and recorded, as well as 5-a reductase inhibitors (5ARIs). The gentleman has continued to work at his bank in his apprenticeship position. He is presently experiencing fatigue and problems when urinating. He has numerous questions about his disease, its evolution, and potential invasive treatment if the low-risk cancer eventually evolves to where aggressive treatment is required. Thus, this gentleman indicates that he is experiencing a lot of anxiety and uncertainty related to his present health status. His spouse is equally unclear about the threat of the disease, its potential evolution and the possibility of invasive treatment.

At the next consultation and screening examination, where the spouse is present, the gentleman is told by the physician that due to his low-risk cancer active surveillance can continue for another 21 months. It is not possible to determine the actual evolution of the disease. The gentleman and his spouse are dismayed and worried. They are fearful of the future due to the uncertain nature of his cancer. The physician tries to provide information about the disease, its evolution and potential outcomes. However, neither the gentleman or his spouse have found the information helpful. They feel more confused and anxious as each minute passes. They would have preferred for anti-cancer treatment to start immediately. To improve the situation and reduce uncertainty experienced by the gentleman and his spouse, the physician proceeded to conduct a thorough assessment of the gentleman's and spouse's uncertainty and anxiety levels. In addition, the physician worked to identify the level of knowledge both the gentleman and his spouse had about the disease. Based on these data, the physician was then able to proceed to carefully explain the disease more fully to both providing pictorial support. After going through adequate material, the physician invited the gentleman and his spouse to re-discuss their perspective of the situation in three months' time rather than wait six months for the next consultation.

In consideration of recommendations within the theory *The Omnipresence of Cancer*, the physician aimed at transparency. By offering a shorter period of waiting until the next consultation, the physician was able to address the fear, anxiety, and uncertainty both the gentleman and his spouse were experiencing and go some way toward reducing their impact on the everyday experience of their lives.

Conclusion

In this chapter, a concept analysis of uncertainty has been presented. It has been identified that uncertainty constitutes an important influencing factor in a patient's cancer trajectory. Therefore, it is recommended integration of regular and systematic assessments from the moment of diagnosis onward, to discern the presence of uncertainty amongst patients and their families. Uncertainty appears to be a factor present in almost any type of cancer, regardless of gender, age, or level of education. Healthcare providers are described as lacking sufficient information on the experience of uncertainty to effectively assist patients undergoing cancer treatments. *The Omnipresence of Cancer*, as a theory, can assist healthcare providers identify the symptoms of uncertainty and understand the importance of how uncertainty affects the patient and family. *The Omnipresence of Cancer*, integrated in care as a theory, will facilitate healthcare providers' support of the development of adequate interventions amongst patients and their families, as well as other healthcare professionals.

References

Al Qadire, M. 2014. Jordanian cancer patients' information needs and information-seeking behaviour: a descriptive study. *European Journal of Oncology Nursing*, 18, 46–51.

Aldaz, B. E., Treharne, G. J., Knight, R. G., Conner, T. S. and Perez, D. 2016. "It gets into your head as well as your body": the experiences of patients with cancer during oncology treatment with curative intent. *Journal of Health Psychology*.

American Cancer Society. 2017. *Cancer Facts and Figures 2017*. Atlanta: American Cancer Society.

Arber, A. and Spencer, L. 2013. "It's all bad news": the first 3 months following a diagnosis of malignant pleural mesothelioma. *Psycho-Oncology*, 22, 1528–33.

Arndt, V., Feller, A., Hauri, D., Heusser, R., Junker, C., Kuehni, C., Lorez, M., Pfeiffer, V., Roy, E. and Schindler, M. 2016. Schweizerischer Krebsbericht 2015. Stand der Entwicklungen. In Bundesamt Für Statistik, Nationales Institut Für Krebsepidemiologie Und -Registrierung (NICER) & Schweizer Kinderkrebsregister (SKKR) (eds.), Neuchâtel: BFS, Gesundheitsorbservatorium.

Bailey, D. E., Jr., Wallace Kazer, M., Latini, D. M., Hegarty, J., Carroll, P. R., Klein, E. A. and Albertsen, P. C. 2011. Measuring illness uncertainty in men undergoing active surveillance for prostate cancer. *Applied Nursing Research*, 24, 193–9.

Bailey, D. E., Jr., Wallace Kazer, M., Polascik, T. J. and Robertson, C. 2014. Psychosocial trajectories of men monitoring prostate-specific antigen levels following surgery for prostate cancer. *Oncology Nursing Forum*, 41, 361–8.

Beach, W. A. and Dozier, D. M. 2015. Fears, uncertainties, and hopes: patient-initiated actions and doctors' responses during oncology interviews. *Journal of Health Communication*, 20, 1243–54.

Beesley, V. L., Janda, M., Goldstein, D., Gooden, H., Merrett, N. D., O'Connell, D. L., Rowlands, I. J., Wyld, D. and Neale, R. E. 2016. A tsunami of unmet needs: pancreatic and ampullary cancer patients' supportive care needs and use of community and allied health services. *Psycho-Oncology*, 25, 150–7.

Black, G., Sheringham, J., Spencer-Hughes, V., Ridge, M., Lyons, M., Williams, C., Fulop, N. and Pritchard-Jones, K. 2015. Patients' experiences of cancer diagnosis as a result of an emergency presentation: a qualitative study. *PLoS One*, 10, e0135027.

Bogaarts, M. P., Den Oudsten, B. L., Roukema, J. A., Van Riel, J. M., Beerepoot, L. V. and De Vries, J. 2012. The Psychosocial Distress Questionnaire-Breast Cancer (PDQ-BC) is a useful instrument to screen psychosocial problems. *Support Care Cancer*, 20, 1659–65.

Brataas, H. V., Thorsnes, S. L. and Hargie, O. 2010. Themes and goals in cancer outpatient-cancer nurse consultations. *European Journal of Cancer Care (England)*, 19, 184–91.

Brown, D. and Oetzel, J. 2016. Men's use of networks to manage communication tensions related to a potential diagnosis of prostate cancer. *European Journal of Oncology Nursing*, 20, 106–12.

Cahill, J., Lobiondo-Wood, G., Bergstrom, N. and Armstrong, T. 2012. Brain tumor symptoms as antecedents to uncertainty: an integrative review. *Journal of Nursing Scholarship*, 44, 145–55.

Campbell-Enns, H. J. and Woodgate, R. L. 2016. The psychosocial experiences of women with breast cancer across the lifespan: a systematic review. *Psycho-Oncology*.

Carlson, L. E. 2016. Mindfulness-based interventions for coping with cancer. *Annals of the New York Academy of Sciences*, 1373, 5–12.

Cavers, D., Hacking, B., Erridge, S. C., Morris, P. G., Kendall, M. and Murray, S. A. 2013. Adjustment and support needs of glioma patients and their relatives: serial interviews. *Psycho-Oncology*, 22, 1299–305.

Checton, M. G., Greene, K., Magsamen-Conrad, K. and Venetis, M. K. 2012. Patients' and spouses' perspectives of chronic illness and its management. *Families, Systems, & Health*, 30, 114–29.

Donovan, M. and Glackin, M. 2012. The lived experience of patients receiving radiotherapy for head and neck cancer: a literature review. *International Journal of Palliative Nursing*, 18, 448–55.

Edib, Z., Kumarasamy, V., Binti Abdullah, N., Rizal, A. M. and Al-Dubai, S. A. 2016. Most prevalent unmet supportive care needs and quality of life of breast cancer patients in a tertiary hospital in Malaysia. *Health and Quality of Life Outcomes*, 14, 26.

Ellis, J., Brearley, S. G., Craven, O. and Molassiotis, A. 2013. Understanding the symptom experience of patients with gastrointestinal cancers in the first year following diagnosis: findings from a qualitative longitudinal study. *Journal of Gastrointestinal Cancer*, 44, 60–7.

Elphee, E. E. 2008. Understanding the concept of uncertainty in patients with indolent lymphoma. *Oncology Nursing Forum*, 35, 449–54.

Ghodraty-Jabloo, V., Alibhai, S. M., Breunis, H. and Puts, M. T. 2016. Keep your mind off negative things: coping with long-term effects of acute myeloid leukemia (AML). *Support Care Cancer*, 24, 2035–45.

Giammanco, M. D., Gitto, L., Barberis, N. and Santoro, D. 2015. Adaptation of the Mishel Uncertainty of Illness Scale (MUIS) for chronic patients in Italy. *Journal of Evaluation in Clinical Practice*, 21, 649–55.

Goh, A. C., Kowalkowski, M. A., Bailey, D. E., Jr., Kazer, M. W., Knight, S. J. and Latini, D. M. 2012. Perception of cancer and inconsistency in medical information are associated with decisional conflict: a pilot study of men with prostate cancer who undergo active surveillance. *BJU International*, 110, E50–6.

Grimsbo, G. H., Finset, A. and Ruland, C. M. 2011. Left hanging in the air: experiences of living with cancer as expressed through E-mail communications with oncology nurses. *Cancer Nursing*, 34, 107–16.

Hagen, K. B., Aas, T., Lode, K., Gjerde, J., Lien, E., Kvaloy, J. T., Lash, T. L., Soiland, H. and Lind, R. 2015. Illness uncertainty in breast cancer patients: validation of the 5-item short form of the Mishel Uncertainty in Illness Scale. *European Journal of Oncology Nursing*, 19, 113–9.

Haisfield-Wolfe, M. E., McGuire, D. B., Soeken, K., Geiger-Brown, J., De Forge, B. and Suntharalingam, M. 2012. Prevalence and correlates of symptoms and uncertainty in illness among head and neck cancer patients receiving definitive radiation with or without chemotherapy. *Support Care Cancer*, 20, 1885–93.

Hall, D. L., Mishel, M. H. and Germino, B. B. 2014. Living with cancer-related uncertainty: associations with fatigue, insomnia, and affect in younger breast cancer survivors. *Support Care Cancer*, 22, 2489–95.

Hammond, C., Reese, M. and Teucher, U. 2015. Tricksterdom in narratives of young adult cancer: performances of uncertainty, subversion, and possibility. *Journal of Health Psychology*, 34, 437–45.

Hanratty, B., Addington-Hall, J., Arthur, A., Cooper, L., Grande, G., Payne, S. and Seymour, J. 2013. What is different about living alone with cancer in older age? A qualitative study of experiences and preferences for care. *BMC Family Practice*, 14, 22.

Hendriksen, E., Williams, E., Sporn, N., Greer, J., Degrange, A. and Koopman, C. 2015. Worried together: a qualitative study of shared anxiety in patients with metastatic non-small cell lung cancer and their family caregivers. *Support Care Cancer*, 23, 1035–41.

Horrill, T. 2016. Active surveillance in prostate cancer: a concept analysis. *Journal of Clinical Nursing*, 25, 1166–72.

Hoth, K. F., Wamboldt, F. S., Ford, D. W., Sandhaus, R. A., Strange, C., Bekelman, D. B. and Holm, K. E. 2015. The social environment and illness uncertainty in chronic obstructive pulmonary disease. *International Journal of Behavioral Medicine*, 22, 223–32.

Jeon, B. H., Choi, M., Lee, J. and Noh, S. H. 2016. Relationships between gastrointestinal symptoms, uncertainty, and perceived recovery in patients with gastric cancer after gastrectomy. *Nursing & Health Sciences*, 18, 23–9.

Jones, C. E., Maben, J., Lucas, G., Davies, E. A., Jack, R. H. and Ream, E. 2015. Barriers to early diagnosis of symptomatic breast cancer: a qualitative study of Black African, Black Caribbean and White British women living in the UK. *BMJ Open*, 5, e006944.

Kazer, M. W., Bailey, D. E., Jr. and Whittemore, R. 2010. Out of the black box: expansion of a theory-based intervention to self-manage the uncertainty associated with active surveillance (AS) for prostate cancer. *Research and Theory for Nursing Practice*, 24, 101–12.

Kazer, M. W., Psutka, S. P., Latini, D. M. and Bailey, D. E., Jr. 2013. Psychosocial aspects of active surveillance. *Current Opinion in Urology*, 23, 273–7.

Kennedy, F., Harcourt, D. and Rumsey, N. 2008. The challenge of being diagnosed and treated for ductal carcinoma in situ (DCIS). *European Journal of Oncology Nursing*, 12, 103–11.

Kennedy, F., Harcourt, D., Rumsey, N. and White, P. 2010. The psychosocial impact of ductal carcinoma in situ (DCIS): a longitudinal prospective study. *Breast*, 19, 382–7.

Kurita, K., Garon, E. B., Stanton, A. L. and Meyerowitz, B. E. 2013. Uncertainty and psychological adjustment in patients with lung cancer. *Psycho-Oncology*, 22, 1396–401.

Kyranou, M., Puntillo, K., Dunn, L. B., Aouizerat, B. E., Paul, S. M., Cooper, B. A., Neuhaus, J., West, C., Dodd, M. and Miaskowski, C. 2014. Predictors of initial levels and trajectories of anxiety in women before and for 6 months after breast cancer surgery. *Cancer Nursing*, 37, 406–17.

Lambert, S. D., Girgis, A., Turner, J., McElduff, P., Kayser, K. and Vallentine, P. 2012. A pilot randomized controlled trial of the feasibility of a self-directed coping skills intervention for couples facing prostate cancer: rationale and design. *Health and Quality of Life Outcomes*, 10, 119.

Lang, H., France, E., Williams, B., Humphris, G. and Wells, M. 2013. The psychological experience of living with head and neck cancer: a systematic review and meta-synthesis. *Psycho-Oncology*, 22, 2648–63.

Lim, S. H., Chan, S. W. and He, H. G. 2015. Patients' experiences of performing self-care of stomas in the initial postoperative period. *Cancer Nursing*, 38, 185–93.

Lin, L., Acquaye, A. A., Vera-Bolanos, E., Cahill, J. E., Gilbert, M. R. and Armstrong, T. S. 2012. Validation of the Mishel's uncertainty in illness scale-brain tumor form (MUIS-BT). *Journal of Neuro-Oncology*, 110, 293–300.

Lin, L., Chiang, H. H., Acquaye, A. A., Vera-Bolanos, E., Gilbert, M. R. and Armstrong, T. S. 2013. Uncertainty, mood states, and symptom distress in patients with primary brain tumors: analysis of a conceptual model using structural equation modeling. *Cancer*, 119, 2796–806.

Lin, L., Chien, L. C., Acquaye, A. A., Vera-Bolanos, E., Gilbert, M. R. and Armstrong, T. S. 2015. Significant predictors of patients' uncertainty in primary brain tumors. *Journal of Neuro-Oncology*, 122, 507–15.

Litzelman, K., Blanch-Hartigan, D., Lin, C. C. and Han, X. 2017. Correlates of the positive psychological byproducts of cancer: role of family caregivers and informational support. *Palliat Support Care*, 1–11.

Mazor, K. M., Beard, R. L., Alexander, G. L., Arora, N. K., Firneno, C., Gaglio, B., Greene, S. M., Lemay, C. A., Robinson, B. E., Roblin, D. W., Walsh, K., Street, R. L., Jr. and Gallagher, T. H. 2013. Patients' and family members' views on patient-centered communication during cancer care. *Psycho-Oncology*, 22, 2487–95.

Mishel, M. H. 2014. Theories of uncertainty in illness. In M. J. Smith and P. R. Liehr (eds.), *Middle Range Theory for Nursing*, third edition. New York, NY: Springer.

Mishel, M. H., Germino, B. B., Lin, L., Pruthi, R. S., Wallen, E. M., Crandell, J. and Blyler, D. 2009. Managing uncertainty about treatment decision making in early stage prostate cancer: a randomized clinical trial. *Patient Education and Counseling*, 77, 349–59.

Mollica, M. A., Underwood, W., 3rd, Homish, G. G., Homish, D. L. and Orom, H. 2016. Spirituality is associated with better prostate cancer treatment decision making experiences. *Journal of Behavioral Medicine*, 39, 161–9.

Morse, J. M., Mitcham, C., Hupcey, J. E. and Tason, M. C. 1996. Criteria for concept evaluation. *Journal of Advanced Nursing*, 24, 385–90.

Newcomb, L. F., Thompson, I. M., Jr., Boyer, H. D., Brooks, J. D., Carroll, P. R., Cooperberg, M. R., Dash, A., Ellis, W. J., Fazli, L., Feng, Z., Gleave, M. E., Kunju, P., Lance, R. S., McKenney, J. K., Meng, M. V., Nicolas, M. M., Sanda, M. G., Simko, J., So, A., Tretiakova, M. S., Troyer, D. A., True, L. D., Vakar-Lopez, F., Virgin, J., Wagner, A. A., Wei, J. T., Zheng, Y., Nelson, P. S., Lin, D. W. and Canary, P. I. 2016. Outcomes of active surveillance for clinically localized prostate cancer in the prospective, multi-institutional canary pass cohort. *Journal of Urology*, 195, 313–20.

Oliffe, J. L., Davison, B. J., Pickles, T. and Mroz, L. 2009. The self-management of uncertainty among men undertaking active surveillance for low-risk prostate cancer. *Qualitative Health Research*, 19, 432–43.

Pacian, A., Kulik, T. B., Pacian, J., Chrusciel, P., Zolnierczuk-Kieliszek, D. and Jarosz, M. J. 2012. Psychosocial aspect of quality of life of Polish women with breast cancer. *Annals of Agricultural and Environmental Medicine*, 19, 509–12.

Parahoo, K., McDonough, S., McCaughan, E., Noyes, J., Semple, C., Halstead, E. J., Neuberger, M. M. and Dahm, P. 2015. Psychosocial interventions for men with prostate cancer: a Cochrane systematic review. *BJU International*, 116, 174–83.

Park, J., Neuman, H. B., Bennett, A. V., Polskin, L., Phang, P. T., Wong, W. D. and Temple, L. K. 2014. Patient expectations of functional outcomes after rectal cancer surgery: a qualitative study. *Diseases of the Colon & Rectum*, 57, 151–7.

Parker, P. A., Alba, F., Fellman, B., Urbauer, D. L., Li, Y., Karam, J. A., Tannir, N., Jonasch, E., Wood, C. G. and Matin, S. F. 2013. Illness uncertainty and quality of life of patients with small renal tumors undergoing watchful waiting: a 2-year prospective study. *European Urology*, 63, 1122–7.

Parker, P. A., Davis, J. W., Latini, D. M., Baum, G., Wang, X., Ward, J. F., Kuban, D., Frank, S. J., Lee, A. K., Logothetis, C. J. and Kim, J. 2016. Relationship between illness uncertainty, anxiety, fear of progression and quality of life in men with favourable-risk prostate cancer undergoing active surveillance. *BJU International*, 117, 469–77.

Rains, S. A. 2014. Health information seeking and the World Wide Web: an uncertainty management perspective. *Journal of Health Communication*, 19, 1296–307.

Rains, S. A. and Tukachinsky, R. 2015a. An examination of the relationships among uncertainty, appraisal, and information-seeking behavior proposed in uncertainty management theory. *Health Communication*, 30, 339–49.

Rains, S. A. and Tukachinsky, R. 2015b. Information seeking in uncertainty management theory: exposure to information about medical uncertainty and information-processing orientation as predictors of uncertainty management success. *Journal of Health Communication*, 20, 1275–86.

Rodgers, B. L. 1989. Concepts, analysis and the development of nursing knowledge: the evolutionary cycle. *Journal of Advanced Nursing*, 14, 330–5.

Sajjadi, M., Rassouli, M., Abbaszadeh, A., Alavi Majd, H. and Zendehdel, K. 2014. Psychometric properties of the Persian version of the Mishel's Uncertainty in Illness Scale in patients with cancer. *European Journal of Oncology Nursing*, 18, 52–7.

Sautier, L. P., Vehling, S. and Mehnert, A. 2014. Assessment of patients' dignity in cancer care: preliminary psychometrics of the German version of the Patient Dignity Inventory (PDI-G). *Journal of Pain and Symptom Management*, 47, 181–8.

Schumm, K., Skea, Z., Mckee, L. and N'Dow, J. 2010. 'They're doing surgery on two people': a meta-ethnography of the influences on couples' treatment decision making for prostate cancer. *Health Expectations*, 13, 335–49.

Shaha, M., Cox, C. L., Talman, K. and Kelly, D. 2008. Uncertainty in breast, prostate, and colorectal cancer: implications for supportive care. *Journal of Nursing Scholarship*, 40, 60–7.

Shaha, M., Pandian, V., Choti, M. A., Stotsky, E., Herman, J. M., Khan, Y., Libonati, C., Pawlik, T. M., Schulick, R. D. and Belcher, A. E. 2010. Transitoriness in cancer patients: a cross-sectional survey of lung and gastrointestinal cancer patients. *Supportive Care in Cancer*, 19, 271–9.

Song, L., Northouse, L. L., Braun, T. M., Zhang, L., Cimprich, B., Ronis, D. L. and Mood, D. W. 2011. Assessing longitudinal quality of life in prostate cancer patients and their spouses: a multilevel modeling approach. *Quality of Life Research*, 20, 371–81.

Stenberg, U., Ruland, C. M., Olsson, M. and Ekstedt, M. 2012. To live close to a person with cancer – experiences of family caregivers. *Social Work in Health Care*, 51, 909–26.

Suzuki, M. 2012. Quality of life, uncertainty, and perceived involvement in decision making in patients with head and neck cancer. *Oncology Nursing Forum*, 39, 541–8.

Syrjala, K. L., Yi, J. C. and Langer, S. L. 2016. Psychometric properties of the Cancer and Treatment Distress (CTXD) measure in hematopoietic cell transplantation patients. *Psycho-Oncology*, 25, 529–35.

Taneja, M. K. 2013. Life style management in head and neck cancer patients. *Indian Journal of Otolaryngology and Head & Neck Surgery*, 65, 289–92.

Torre, L. A., Bray, F., Siegel, R. L., Ferlay, J., Lortet-Tieulent, J. and Jemal, A. 2015. Global cancer statistics, 2012. *CA: A Cancer Journal for Clinicians*, 65, 87–108.

Turkman, Y. E., Kennedy, H. P., Harris, L. N. and Knobf, M. T. 2016. "An addendum to breast cancer": the triple negative experience. *Support Care Cancer*, 24, 3715–21.

Watson, M., Davolls, S., Mohammed, K. and Shepherd, S. 2015. The influence of life stage on supportive care and information needs in cancer patients: does older age matter? *Support Care Cancer*, 23, 2981–8.

WHO. 2017. *Fact Sheet. Cancer* [Online]. Geneva: World Health Organization. Available at: www.who.int/mediacentre/factsheets/fs297/en/index.html#. [Accessed February 25, 2017].

Witham, G., Willard, C., Ryan-Woolly, B. and O'Dwyer, S. T. 2008. A study to explore the patient's experience of peritoneal surface malignancies: pseudomyxoma peritonei. *European Journal of Oncology Nursing*, 12, 112–9.

Wong, J. C., Payne, A. Y., Mah, K., Lebel, S., Lee, R. N., Irish, J., Rodin, G. and Devins, G. M. 2013. Negative cancer stereotypes and disease-specific self-concept in head and neck cancer. *Psycho-Oncology*, 22, 1055–63.

Zhang, Y., Kwekkeboom, K. and Petrini, M. 2015. Uncertainty, self-efficacy, and self-care behavior in patients with breast cancer undergoing chemotherapy in China. *Cancer Nursing*, 38, E19–26.

9 Spirituality in healthcare provision

C. Cox

Introduction

The purpose of this chapter is to consider spirituality within the context of healthcare provision. The context of spirituality in healthcare will be addressed sociologically and theologically. It will be argued that nursing, as a practice discipline, has fallen short in relation to discerning an evidence-base for the provision of spiritual care. It will further be shown that although nurses, as healthcare professionals, are credited with initially having nurtured the interest in spirituality and its implications for spiritual care there is profound criticism of its poorly constructed scholarship including conceptual confusion and lack of evidence to substantiate its practice recommendations and claims associated with spiritual care. This then, will be drawn into a parallel of caring for the patient's and or family's spiritual needs, in particular, when the patient and family perceive the patient may be nearing or at the end of life. In this chapter, it will be shown that spiritual care provision can be nourished through an understanding of the theory *The Omnipresence of Cancer* (Shaha and Cox, 2003) and how it informs practice. It will be postulated that *The Omnipresence of Cancer*, as a theory, can be for nurses and healthcare professionals, in general, the beginning of an evidence-base for the delivery of spiritual care.

Presently, in healthcare, there is an indication that nurses and healthcare professionals in general, are unable to substantiate their practice base in relation to spirituality. Although much is written about spiritual care, there appears to be only a small evidence base for the practice of spiritual care within the context of caring for patients nearing or at the end of life. Subsequently nurses, and healthcare professionals (again, in general), are not fulfilling their essential role in caring for the spiritual needs of cancer patients nearing or at the end of life. *The Omnipresence of Cancer* (Shaha and Cox, 2003) provides a foundation for the delivery of spiritual care situated within a sociological and theological context of practice.

Background

Sociological and theological context of practice

The place where sociology and theology 'rub up against each other' is 'in the field of practice' (Sweeney, 2012: 1). Each is in service to people experiencing uncertainty in relation to the transitory nature of life. This is no more evident than when one is facing the end of life. Nursing, as a practice discipline, is intimately involved in the provision of care to people experiencing uncertainty and anxiety within the context of living and dying. The provision of spiritual care features heavily when caring for the sick, particularly so in instances of end of life care. Sweeney (2012: 17) proposes that 'Spirituality is a much discussed feature of contemporary culture and an obvious place to look for sociological-theological convergence. As an emergent sociological construct spirituality is commonly seen in disjunction from "religion".' It has 'migrated from the world of faith, first into theological obscurity, and then into postmodern culture'. Sweeney (2012: 17) notes that 'spirituality is rooted in and constituted from personal experience, sometimes communal experience but more typically the "deep experiences of the self".' It is the deep 'lived experience' (Collins, 2000: 12); particularly in relation to finitude (refer to Chapter 4, *The Omnipresence of Cancer.*) and end of life care that nursing is most concerned. In relation to finitude, there is a sociological and theological convergence associated with spirituality that the nurse should be cognizant of when caring for the patient and family as the end of life nears.

Spirituality, a sociological and theological convergence

According to the Collins English Dictionary (2014), spirituality is identified as relating to the spirit or soul and not physical nature or matter. It is intangible. It relates to sacred things, the Church, religion and standing in a relationship based on communication between souls or minds such as a 'spiritual father' (Collins English Dictionary, 2014: 1298). This perspective is substantiated from an encyclopedic definition in which spirituality is seen as entailing a sense of connection to something greater than oneself (Chao et al., 2002; Wai Man, 2007). The term spirituality is widely used throughout the Western world and, as shown in the Collins English Dictionary (2014), is being understood in varying ways. Its construct is both sociological and theological. It may be considered by the sociologist to denote a religion, faith or practice and to the theologian as faith, a way of being in the world (Augustine, 425; Metz, 1998a, 1998b; Bloom, 1999a, 1999b; Collins, 2000; McGrath, 2000). When defining spirituality, it is apparent that its meaning is elusive and depends on individual perspectives (Wai Man, 2007). Spirituality has further been defined as the search for existential or ultimate meaning within a life experience, such as illness (Speck et al., 2004; Wai Man, 2007). Nursing academia frequently associates spirituality in nursing practice with caring. It is an activity, a way of being with patients. The context of caring involves assisting patients who 'are either sick or well' in the undertaking of their daily activities and 'contributing to their health or recovery or to a peaceful death' (Henderson, 1966: 15). In this sense, spirituality concerns the activity of nourishing the patient's spirit. Nurses view caring for the patient as a moral imperative or ideal (Watson, 1995) and that it involves ministrations which are person-centred, protective, anticipatory, physically comforting and go beyond the routine care of the patient (Watson, 1995; Cox, 2007). It may be viewed that nurses, and all healthcare professionals for that matter, have a moral obligation to ensure that not only the physiological and psychological needs of the patient are met but that the spiritual needs of patient are met as well (Cox, 2007). Spiritual care then, speaks to those who are seeking meaning within the context of their illness, peace within the chaos of their healthcare experience, and light within what they perceive to be a dark and uncertain future. Only too often, this future is seen by patients nearing or at the end of their life as a life that it is filled with suffering.

Suffering

Metz (1998a, 1998b) addresses the issue of suffering and dignity in his writings *On The Way To A Postidealist Theology* and *The Theological Dignity of Humankind.* He references the perspective of Karl Rahner (Refer additionally to the reflection: McNichol's *Reflection on the Spiritual Writings of Karl Rahner, 2011.*) and raises the question (rather abstractly): do we not all feel and live within a time of suffering? A sense is raised to have respect for the dignity of human beings and their experiences of suffering that have (throughout evolution) occurred. There is a call to understand the nature of suffering. His writings converge into an unspoken message to minister (care for) to those who suffer. Within the context of ministering Tyler (2012: 209) considers spiritual direction, once again, from an evolutionary perspective. In the Western world, which is primarily Christian, spiritual direction most often occurs within a 'faith context'. It 'assumes a shared faith' (Tyler, 2012: 209) between the people involved. Nursing and its practice resonate with this view (Cox, 2007). In healthcare, the nurse comes to the patient and and/or their family seeing them in anguish, searching for answers; hoping to find an ultimate healing either through technology or a miracle. Human beings, reach out to a spiritual base for living (Kurtz and Ketcham, 2002). In spiritual care, for patients and their families, a holy place becomes palpable. It is a place where the Creator is often called upon; most discernably at the end of life. It "is a place where human beings discover each other in a caring relationship" (Sellner, 1990; Wai Man, 2007). However, there is a concern here. As previously indicated in this chapter, spiritual care is poorly constructed in its scholarship and there is conceptual confusion regarding the nature of spiritual care.

Spiritual care: poorly constructed scholarship and conceptual confusion

The Department of Health (2010) commissioned a systematic review of the literature on end of life care in which spirituality was addressed. The purpose of the review was to support implementation of the Department of Health's *End of Life Care Strategy* (DoH, 2010) in which guidance is provided on the provision of high-quality spiritual care appropriate to the varying contexts of end of life care in the United Kingdom. In the review 248 sources from 17 different countries were discovered, classified and critically reviewed. It is notable that of the sources, 41% were published in the United Kingdom and 35% were published in the United States. Amongst these were seven collaborative publications between the United Kingdom and the United States. Evidence of the knowledge and tools available for providing spiritual care was gathered. Significant gaps in knowledge and skills (application of intervention models) and considerable practice issues emerged from the findings. Following the review, three consultation groups of academics, practitioners and service users and carers convened to contemplate the findings. In particular, the consultation groups noted that the highest number of publications addressing spirituality were derived from nursing. They also found that although nursing is credited with initially having nurtured the interest in spirituality and its implications for spiritual care there is profound criticism of its poorly constructed scholarship including conceptual confusion and lack of evidence to substantiate its practice recommendations and claims. Furthermore, even though the review found a substantial amount of literature that is relevant to spiritual care at the end of life, there is minimal literature that addresses the context related to end of life spiritual care. The Department of Health report (DoH, 2010) based on the literature and recommendations from the consultation groups indicates that the evidence base for spiritual care requires strengthening, an evaluation of practice models should be undertaken and the education and training of nurses with a specific 'focus on translating academic concepts and theoretical models into accessible practice understandings and viable interventions' must be undertaken (DoH, 2010: 33). One such model that has the potential to substantiate an evidence base for spiritual care is the middle range theory: *The Omnipresence of Cancer* (Shaha and Cox, 2003).

Discussion

Relevance of the theory, The Omnipresence of Cancer in healthcare provision

You will recall that in Chapter 4, *The Omnipresence of Cancer*, there are two dimensions: *Toward Authentic Dasein* and *Mapping Out the Future*. Within the dimensions of *Toward Authentic Dasein* and *Mapping Out the Future*, the constructs of Transitoriness and Uncertainty are featured. Although *The Omnipresence of Cancer*, as a theory, does not directly articulate a spiritual construct, the nature of spirituality can be deduced from narrative associated with Transitoriness and Uncertainty and ultimately the human being's view of Finitude (Shaha and Cox, 2003; Heidegger, 1962). In Chapter 2 of this monograph, an ontological view of the human being is seen as Dasein. A conclusion can be drawn from Heidegger's (1962) premise associated with Dasein that any theory based on a foundation of *Being in Time* (Heidegger, 1962) would have within it assumptions relating to the support of Dasein spiritually. It is contended that spiritual support of the patient and family is critically in need as the healthcare environment becomes more mechanized and secular in its approach to caring and care (refer to Chapter 2). The phenomenological world view in *Being in Time* (Heidegger, 1962) presents the foundation for a spiritual dimension in *The Omnipresence of Cancer* (Shaha and Cox, 2003). Perhaps this is most indicative in the theory's construct *Mapping Out the Future*. Penetration of the theory into the minds and hearts of nurses can influence how they approach patients and their families and how they assist patients and their families in their need to map out their future when their future seems uncertain and transitory. For example, in "Coming Full Circle, Doulas Now Cradle the Dying" (Kaiser Health News, Pensacola News Journal, 2017) it is shown that Doulas[1] (originally a Greek word for a woman helping another woman, which is now nurses, doctors and other healthcare professionals as well as specially trained male and female volunteers) support patients at the end of life by fulfilling patients' wishes through the provision of spiritual care. Spiritual care goes beyond a focus on physical needs. In spiritual care, Doulas help the dying reflect on life's meaning and conduct comforting rituals, such as light touch massage and holding hands. Reading to patients and playing the patient's favorite music and or singing with patients facilitates relaxation. Doulas also explain signs and symptoms of dying to family members and help them to know what is coming next in the dying process.

The healthcare environment can become one in which nurses, when utilizing the theory *The Omnipresence of Cancer*, can present a new way of being (like Doulas present) with patients and their families in the everydayness of their practice and particularly when engaged in end of life care. In light of the aforementioned, a case study is presented in the narrative that follows. Its intention is to demonstrate how *The Omnipresence of Cancer*, as a theory, can inform practice.

Case example for practice

In Chapter 4, a case study is presented in which the patient experiences uncertainty and contemplates the transitory nature of her life. Aspects of the case study are presented here and related to the need for and provision of spiritual care. Aspects of the case study in Chapter 4 are quoted, and suggestions are given for spiritual care within constructs inherent in *The Omnipresence of Cancer*. These are, namely, Transitoriness, Uncertainty and Finitude.

Day 1

Oh Gott, the vomiting won't stop. My insides are spilling out of my mouth. The taste is foul and this Furcht und Angst are all consuming. It is unglaublich! The vomiting won't stop . . . won't stop. Oh Gott, help me . . . help me. Warum ich? Warum ich? (In this narrative, it is evident that the patient is calling on a higher power to help her. As the patient calls out, the nurse can support the patient and family by discerning through dialogue with the patient and family if they have a faith-based belief in a creator, if the patient would like to receive visits from a chaplain of their faith or would like someone else to speak with about their concerns and fears. Not allowing the patient to go without the administration of adequate medication to alleviate the vomiting will promote comfort so that the patient can rest and the family can see that the patient is comfortable. Once the patient is comfortable the potential for the patient and family to receive visitors who can facilitate meeting their spiritual needs becomes possible.)

Day 26

I'm dying . . . Yes, it is probably so. I've seen my face. I can't look at it any more. The lines . . . I've lost my hair. I am no longer the same. The ugly growth that they cut from me is on the outside now. It shows in my eyes, my skin and the bag on my belly . . . it is foul . . . foul. It is the Chemotherapie und Darmkrebs . . . they are killing me! (In this narrative, it is evident that the patient is perceiving her life is ending. Spiritual support can be provided by the nurse being present with the patient. It involves care that is unhurried and spending time with the patient and family. This may be by sitting quietly at the bedside for a period of time, holding the patient's hand, providing light touch massage and/or offering to pray with the patient if the patient has a faith base or asks for the nurse to pray with her. The nurse can contact the hospital chaplain and alert the chaplain to the patient's need for spiritual support. If the patient does not have a faith base, assisting (or teaching) the patient to meditate can alleviate feelings of anxiety and provide a spiritual grounding in which the patient becomes in touch with herself. Being present involves openness; therefore, the nurse should encourage the patient to talk about her feelings and fears and be receptive to the patient's and family's perspective.)

Day 33

Where is my future? I can't imagine any kind of future . . . not anymore. What about the trip my husband and I were going to take next year? If I live, will I be able to travel at all? How will it be? Will he want me with this scar on my belly and this bag? How can he stand to look at me now? I can't stand to look at myself. I'm ugly . . . this thing is hideous! I might be dead in a year. What does it matter now?

Warum ich? Warum ich? Why does this thing stay with me? Always there. What have I done wrong? (In this narrative, it is evident that the patient is uncertain about her future. Encouraging the doctor to discuss the prognosis openly with the patient and the nurse being willing to discuss the cancer diagnosis and prognosis provides assurance in what to expect. Encouraging the patient and family to talk about their plans and providing a schedule of activities that the patient can review daily provides a sense of certainty about what the patient can expect next. The schedule assists in providing concreteness to daily activities. The schedule should incorporate regular visiting times for the patient's family and chaplain. If the patient has a faith base, incorporating times in the schedule to pray and rest will be important to the patient and family. If the patient does not have a faith base, encouraging meditation at regularly scheduled times can facilitate introspection and a feeling of peace. These are activities in which the patient can look forward. In relation to *Mapping Out the Future*, the nurse should encourage the patient and her husband to begin making plans for activities the two of them will engage in once the patient leaves the hospital. Activities between the patient and her husband can also be incorporated into care provision whilst the patient is in hospital. The patient perceives she is ugly and must have done something 'wrong' and subsequently has contracted cancer. It is important for the nurse in these situations to reassure the patient that her husband wants to be with her. She has not done anything wrong that has brought about the cancer. In conclusion, further contemplation of the theory *The Omnipresence of Cancer* in Chapter 4 can assist the nurse and healthcare provider to understand more fully how to support the spiritual needs of patients and their families.

Conclusion

This chapter has postulated that nursing and in general healthcare as practice disciplines have yet to find their way in relation to discerning an evidence-base for the provision of spiritual care. It has been shown that although nursing is credited with initially having nurtured the interest in spirituality and its implications for spiritual care, there is profound criticism of its poorly constructed scholarship, including conceptual confusion and lack of evidence to substantiate its practice recommendations and claims associated with spiritual care. Indeed, it is evident that nurses and healthcare professionals, in general, are unable to substantiate their practice base in regard to spirituality and do not have a definitive evidence base for the practice of spiritual care, particularly within the context of end-of-life care. Subsequently, nurses and healthcare professionals in general are not presently fulfilling their essential role in caring for the spiritual needs of patients nearing or at the end of life.

Research indicates that social support and improved dyadic communication reduce uncertainty in cancer patients and their partners (Song et al., 2011). Issues regarding the medical treatment plan, the disease situation including the prognosis and patients' psychosocial responses to the disease constitute important areas of communciation between healthcare professionals and patients. These are important issues to consider when rendering spiritual care.

Spiritual care is a critical component of practice according to the systematic review of the literature (*Spiritual Care at the End of Life: a systematic review of the literature*) commissioned by the Department of Health in 2010. It is postulated that this is especially true in relation to end of life care that addresses the spiritual needs of patients and their families. *The Omnipresence of Cancer*, as a theory, can be for nurses and healthcare professionals, in general, the beginning of an evidence base for the delivery of spiritual care.

Note

1 The National Hospice and Palliative Care Organization supports the end-of-life Doula movement ("Coming Full Circle, Doulas Now Cradle the Dying", Kaiser Health News, 2017 in the Pensacola News Journal, 2017.)

References

Augustine, St. Aurelii, ed. 2005. *(425 AD) De Civitate Dei* (The City of God), Books 1 and 2, trans. by P.G. Walsh. Oxford: Oxbow Books.

Bloom, Metropolitan Anthony of Sourozh, ed. 1999a. *School for Prayer.* London: Darton, Longman and Todd Ltd.

Bloom, Metropolitan Anthony of Sourozh, ed. 1999b. *Living Prayer.* London: Darton, Longman and Todd Ltd.

Chao, C., Chen. C. and Yen, M. 2002. The essence of spirituality of terminally ill patients. *Journal of Nursing Research*, 10, 237–44.

Collins. 2014. *Collins English Dictionary 2014.* Glasgow: Harper Collins Publishers, p. 1298.

Collins, Kennith J. 2000. Introduction. In *Exploring Christian Spirituality and Ecumenical Reader*, ed. by K. J. Collins. Grand Rapids: Baker Books, p. 12.

Cox, C. L. 2007. Introduction. In *Caring for the Catholic Patient, Meeting the Pastoral Needs of Catholic Patients*, ed. by The Catholic Bishops' Conference of England and Wales. London: Catholic Truth Society, pp. 3–5.

Department of Health. 2010. *Spiritual Care at the End of Life: A Systematic Review of the Literature.* London: Department of Health, p. 33.

Heidegger, M. 1962. *Being and Time*, trans. by J. Macquarrie and E. Robinson. Oxford: Basil Blackwell Ltd, reprint of the first edition of 1962.

Henderson, Virginia, ed. 1966. *The Nature of Nursing.* New York: Macmillan Publishing, p. 15.

Kaiser Health News. 2017. Coming full circle, doulas now cradle the dying, *Pensacola News Journal*, p. 9B.

Kurtz, E. and Ketcham, K. 2002. *The Spirituality of Imperfection.* New York: Bantam Books.

McGrath, A. E. 2000. Theological foundations for spirituality: basic issues. In Alister E. McGrath (ed.), *Christian Spirituality.* Oxford: Blackwell Publishers, pp. 25–34.

McNichol, H. 2011. *Reflections on the Spiritual Writings of Karl Rahner*. Available at: www.academia.edu/982816/Reflection_on_Spiritual_Writings_of_Karl_Rahner

Metz, J. B. 1998a. On the way to a postidealist theology. In J. Matthew Ashley (trans. and ed.), *Johann Baptist Metz: A Passion for God the Mystical-Political Dimension of Christianity*. New York: Paulist Press, pp. 30–53.

Metz, J. B. 1998b. The theological dignity of humankind. In J. Matthew Ashley (trans. and ed.), *Johann Baptist Metz: A Passion for God The Mystical-Political Dimension of Christianity*. New York: Paulist Press, pp. 107–20.

Sellner, E. 1990. *Mentoring: The Ministry of Spiritual Kinship*. Notre Dame: Ave Maria Press.

Shaha, M. and Cox, C. L. 2003. The omnipresence of cancer. *European Journal of Oncology Nursing*, 7, 191–6.

Song, L., Northouse, L. L., Braun, T. M., Zhang, L., Cimprich, B., Ronis, D. L. and Mood, D. W. 2011. Assessing longitudinal quality of life in prostate cancer patients and their spouses: a multilevel modeling approach. *Qual Life Res*, 20, 371–81.

Speck, P., Higginson, I. and Addington-Hall, J. 2004. Spiritual needs in health care. *British Medical Journal*, 329, 123–4.

Sweeney, J. 2012. Theology & sociology. In Gavin D'Costa and Peter Hampson (eds.), *Christianity and the Disciplines: The Transformation of the University*. London: Continuum. Available at: http://publications.heythrop.ac.uk/1445/ (Accessed November 27, 2012).

Tyler, P. 2012. Christian spiritual direction. In Richard Woods and Peter Tyler (eds.), *The Bloombsury Guide to Christian Spirituality*. London: Bloomsbury, pp. 200–13.

Wai Man, L. 2007. *Spiritual Care Approaches in Death and Dying*. 4th Hong Kong Palliative Care Symposium. Hong Kong: HKSPM Newsletter April & August Issue, pp. 22–5.

Watson, J. ed. 1995. *Nursing: Human Science and Human Care*. Norwalk: Appleton-Century Crofts.

10 Epilogue

C. Cox and M. Zumstein-Shaha

Introduction

In this monograph, the theory *The Omnipresence of Cancer* has been articulated. This theory is original. It emerged from doctoral research undertaken by Maya Shaha under the supervision of Professor Carol Lynn Cox at City University London. Since the construction of the theory, further research has been conducted based on the theory's concepts. Most of these studies have been undertaken in nursing. However, as this monograph demonstrates, the theory is broader in reach than nursing and has relevance for other healthcare professions involved in caring for patients with life-threatening and chronic diseases.

Background

The Omnipresence of Cancer derived its beginning in a qualitative study that employed a phenomenological research design based on Heidegger's Ontology of Dasein[1] (Shaha, 2003; Shaha and Cox, 2003). Following construction of the theory, five preliminary studies employing qualitative and quantitative designs were conducted to further develop the theory and substantiate its scientific basis. In theory-building order, the first four were: two concept analyses exploring the concepts Uncertainty (Shaha et al., 2008) and Transitoriness (Shaha et al., 2011a), a secondary thematic analysis to further explore the concept of Transitoriness (Shaha and Bauer-Wu, 2009) and a cross-sectional study that explored the associations between the concepts of Uncertainty, Transitoriness, Control and Quality of life (Shaha et al., 2010). The series of studies concluded with an exploration of the contribution of the concept analyses to nursing science (Shaha et al., 2011b). Subsequent to the aforementioned research, Bachelor's Degree, Master's Degree and Doctoral Degree research projects have been conducted. Each of these expand and further substantiate the scientific nature of the theory. The purpose of the theory *The Omnipresence of Cancer* is to facilitate an understanding of having been diagnosed with cancer and its effect on the ontology[2] of human existence multi-dimensionally.

Discussion

To date, this theory is employed in Bachelor of Nursing Education and research by Sandra Gaillard Desmedt, one of the co-authors of a chapter in this monograph. The theory is introduced to Baccalaureate students to identify oncological patients' needs and to determine adequate nursing interventions. The theory is also used as frame of reference for research at Master's in Nursing and Doctorate in Nursing Programs. The co-authors, Sandra Gaillard Desmedt, Gora DaRocha and Gina Tavares Sobral have conducted advanced degree studies based on the theory. *The Omnipresence of Cancer* has served as a frame of reference for the theoretical foundation of their research. Their research is presented in this monograph. Several other studies have been conducted and are currently being conducted at Master's Degree level, utilizing the theory as a frame of reference and theoretical foundation. Similarly, the theory has been used a frame of reference for Doctoral research in nursing by Gora DaRocha (another chapter co-author) and Jelena Stanic. In her Doctoral research, Gora DaRocha has developed a life-review intervention. The life-review intervention has been tested for its feasibility of use with patients having advanced cancer disease. Jelena Stanic has initiated Doctoral research, using the theory as a theoretical foundation for determining the psychometric properties of the instrument that measures the experience of Transitoriness. Several Master's Degree studies are associated with this endeavor, notably by Josepha Pasche, Cédric Bussy and Anne-Claude Chaudhry-Schaer. Gina Tavares Sobral (co-author of a chapter in this monograph) has conducted the first step in this endeavor.

Conclusion

In the future, it is planned to explore the experience and expectations of spirituality with patients who are newly diagnosed with cancer and a close family member. It is also planned to further explore dimensions of *The Omnipresence of Cancer* (such as Toward Authentic Dasein and Mapping Out the Future) within patient populations that suffer from chronic diseases. Ultimately, the theory will be expanded to provide perspectives on associated care, assessment instruments for the identification of patient perceptions of their illness and necessitated caring interventions.

Notes

1 Dasein is a German word that means "being there" or "presence".
2 Ontology means specification of a conceptualization.

References

Shaha, M. 2003. *The Omnipresence of Cancer*. Doctoral thesis, City University London.

Shaha, M. and Bauer-Wu, S. 2009. Early adulthood uprooted: transitoriness in young women with breast cancer. *Cancer Nursing*, 32, 246–55.

Shaha, M. and Cox, C. L. 2003. The omnipresence of cancer. *European Journal of Oncology Nursing*, 7, 191–6.

Shaha, M., Cox, C. L., Belcher, A. E. and Cohen, M. Z. 2011a. Transitoriness: patients' perception of life after a diagnosis of cancer. *Cancer Nursing Practice*, 10, 24–7.

Shaha, M., Cox, C. L., Cohen, M. Z., Belcher, A. E. and Kappeli, S. 2011b. The contribution of concept development to nursing knowledge? The example of transitoriness. *Pflege*, 24, 361–72.

Shaha, M., Cox, C. L., Talman, K. and Kelly, D. 2008. Uncertainty in breast, prostate, and colorectal cancer: implications for supportive care. *Journal of Nursing Scholarship*, 40, 60–7.

Shaha, M., Pandian, V., Choti, M. A., Stotsky, E., Herman, J. M., Khan, Y., Libonati, C., Pawlik, T. M., Schulick, R. D. and Belcher, A. E. 2010. Transitoriness in cancer patients: a cross-sectional survey of lung and gastrointestinal cancer patients. *Supportive Care in Cancer*, 19, 271–9.

Index

Page numbers in italic indicate a figure and page numbers in bold indicate a table on the corresponding page.